ESSENCE
and
EMBER

German original title: Heilsames Räuchern: Balsam für die Seele - Mit heimischen Kräutern, Harzen und Hölzern

Copyright © 2022 by original publisher, HEEL Verlag GmbH, Königswinter
Original German edition project management: Christine Birnbaum
Original German edition design: Sabine Vonderstein, Cologne
Translated from the German by David Johnston

English-language edition published by © 2024 Schiffer Publishing

Library of Congress Control Number: 2024932157

Type set in: Bree/Champagne & Limousines
Cover design by: Danielle Farmer
ISBN: 978-0-7643-6752-6
Printed in China

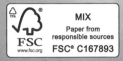

Published by Schiffer Publishing, Ltd.
4880 Lower Valley Road
Atglen, PA 19310
Phone: (610) 593-1777; Fax: (610) 593-2002
Email: info@schifferbooks.com
Web: www.schifferbooks.com

For our complete selection of fine books on this and related subjects, please visit our website at www.schifferbooks.com. You may also write for a free catalog.

Schiffer Publishing's titles are available at special discounts for bulk purchases for sales promotions or premiums. Special editions, including personalized covers, corporate imprints, and excerpts, can be created in large quantities for special needs. For more information, contact the publisher.

Images © Katja Peters, except for:

© adobe.stock.com: page 80: © Dagmar Gärtner, pages 110/111: © Robert Knapp, © k_samurkas, page 118: © sabyna75, page 125: © Nicolas St-Germain

Illustrations: Flowers, Designed by Kjpargeter/Freepik; Watercolour, © chyworks/shutterstock

page 9: Mint Tacuinum sanitates (Minze Tacuinum sanitates) 1380-1399/ Austrian National Library, page 8: Rue Tacuinum sanitates (Weinraute Tacuinum sanitates) 1380-1399/ Austrian National Library.

Disclaimer: This book and the preparations contained therein have been written to the best of our knowledge and belief. Neither the publisher nor the author is responsible for any adverse reactions, consequences, or impairments that may arise from the foraging, identification, growing, processing, or use of the ingredients. In some locations, the plants included here may have a protected status. Check with local regulations before harvesting any wild plants.

Katja Peters

ESSENCE
and
EMBER

Gathering and Preparing Herbal,
Resin, and Wood Incense

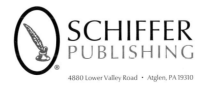

SCHIFFER
PUBLISHING

4880 Lower Valley Road • Atglen, PA 19310

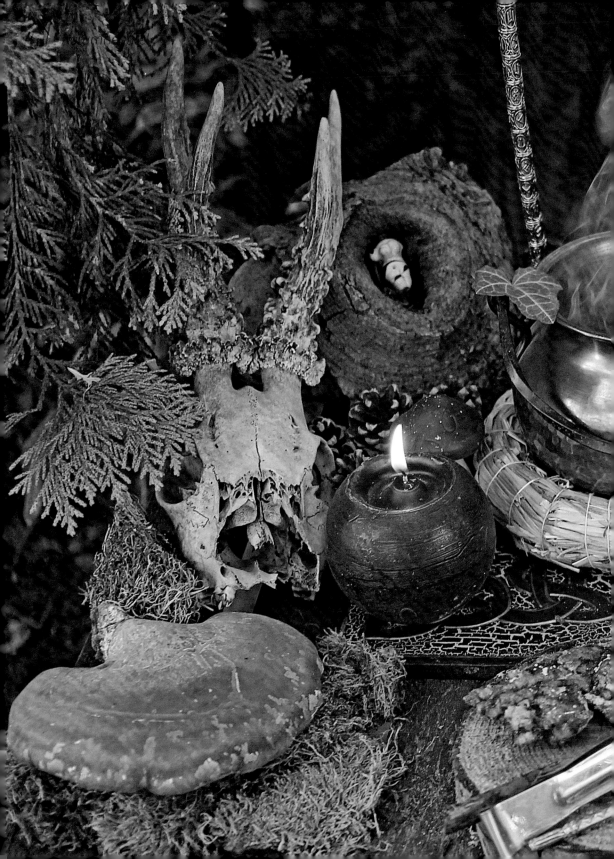

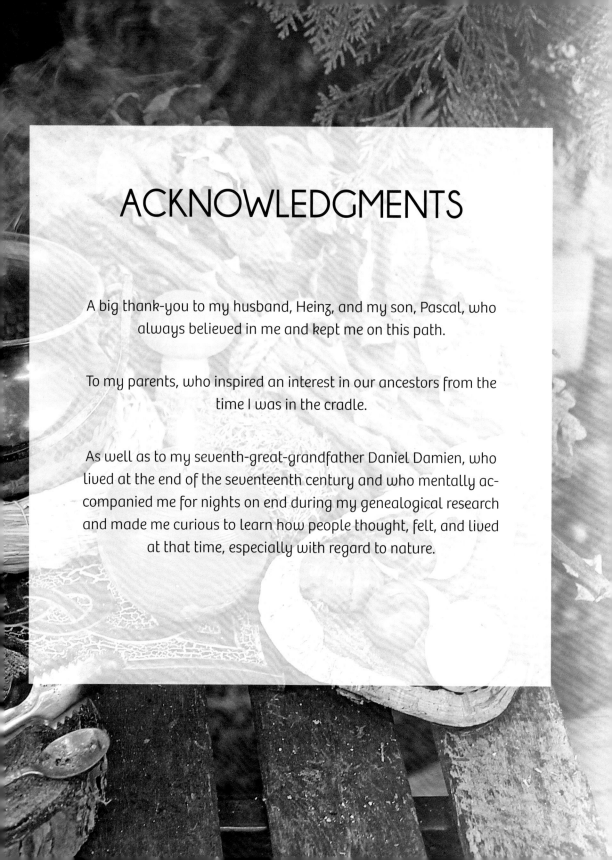

ACKNOWLEDGMENTS

A big thank-you to my husband, Heinz, and my son, Pascal, who always believed in me and kept me on this path.

To my parents, who inspired an interest in our ancestors from the time I was in the cradle.

As well as to my seventh-great-grandfather Daniel Damien, who lived at the end of the seventeenth century and who mentally accompanied me for nights on end during my genealogical research and made me curious to learn how people thought, felt, and lived at that time, especially with regard to nature.

CONTENTS

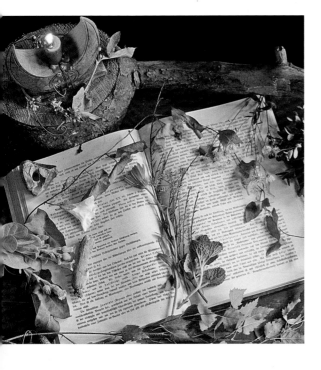

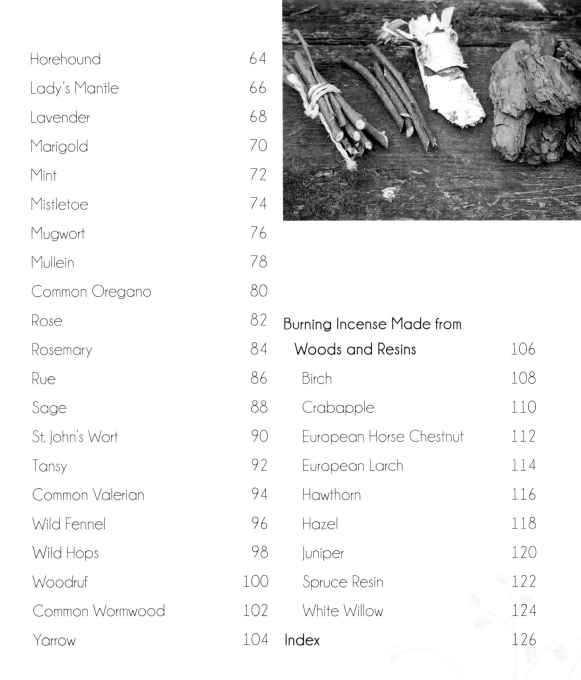

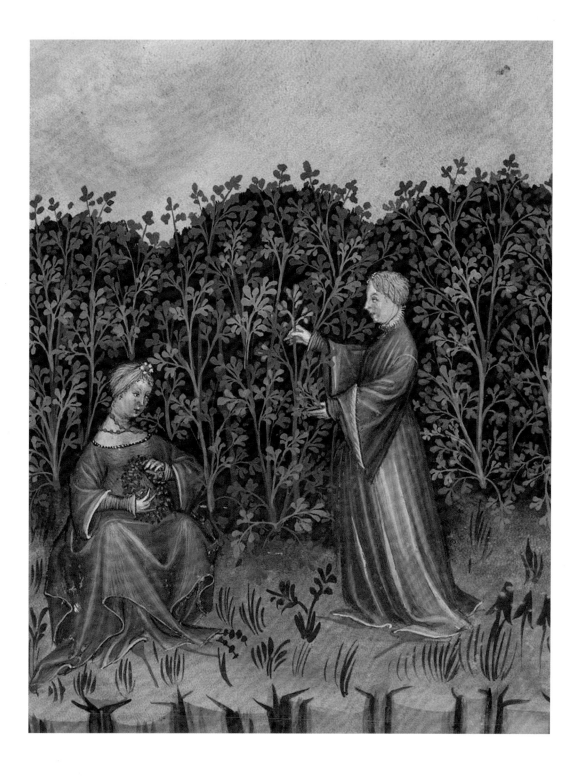

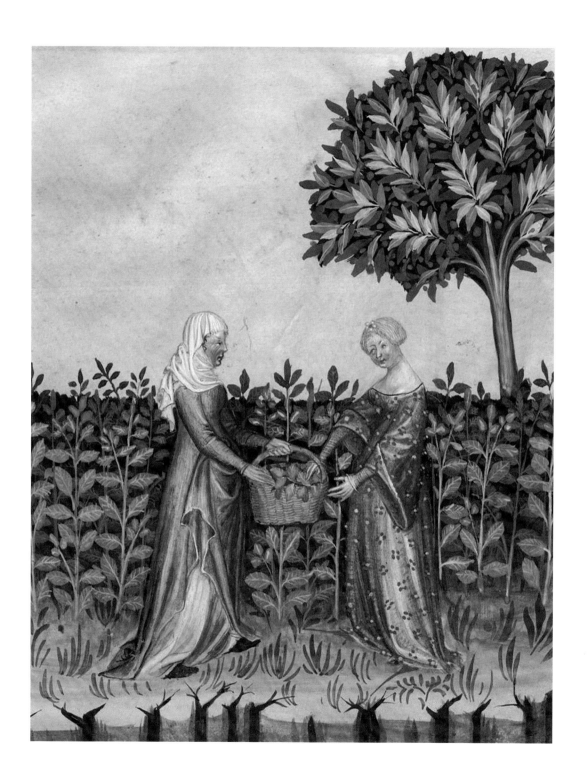

FOREWORD

The burning of incense made from plants has always exerted a fascination on us humans. This is especially true today for us, who live rationally and to whom folk beliefs are foreign. To our ancestors it was customary and completely normal to ward off illnesses, storms, and all sorts of damage to home and property by burning incense.

I have written this book to teach you about the German tradition of burning incense made from herbs, resins, and woods, because my blog has made me realize just how many questions there are in this area. Therefore, I have attempted, as always, to explain the respective topics with short and concise descriptions.

Each incense plant has a message, which is transmitted to us when we burn the incense made from it, because incense lore has also evolved according to the pulse of the time. Nowadays it is important to us to find (inner) peace and to resolve conflicts with people. We are unable to identify with the hardships and fears of our ancestors; nevertheless, our current practices with incense have their origins in the incense lore of old.

Therefore, we should never disregard this history in our own use of incenses, since we can see many parallels in it.

I am very inspired by the eighteenth century. It was followed by the Enlightenment, and folk beliefs slowly disappeared from the population. This occurred more quickly in the city than in the countryside, where people still frequently burned incense and believed in ghosts, demons, and witches. One can see depression, diseases, and negative energies as the modern equivalents of these three "figures."

When I refer to "our ancestors," as a German citizen, I am referring to my own German ancestors, as this book is a window into my culture and written from my perspective; however, I also refer to European roots in general. Because these incense plants were used not only in Germany but also in England, France, Ireland, and in the Scandinavian countries. I hope that this book can spark interest not only in Europe and North America, but worldwide, regardless of one's nationality or heritage.

Many of the presented incense plants not only grow in Germany but also in other European countries. Additionally, in North America, as well as many other parts of the globe, we find many of these same wild plants. Many of these plants migrated to North America with my German ancestors a long time ago and can be harvested in nature there, such as St. John's Wort, which found its home there in 1793, or horehound, which has long been naturalized there. Whatever country you reside in, check with your local botany and ecology organizations and authorities/regulations to determine the accessibility and protection status of these plants.

Some European-species incense plants listed in this book can be replaced with their native versions, such as sage or mistletoe. As for sage, this beautiful and very powerful plant has always had a banishing property against negative energies worldwide. It is also used for fumigations in old houses. Therefore, any form of sage can be used for smoking. In North

America, for example, it is White Sage that was used by Indigenous peoples for these purposes. Now let's take European Goldenrod, which can be wonderfully replaced with Canadian Goldenrod, native to North America. Just be sure to check with your local wildlife authorities to determine the legality of harvesting and the safety of burning any and all plants. Many may find it simpler to cultivate one's own incense garden with plants bought from purveyors.

In ancient smoking practices, there are many parallels among ancient peoples worldwide. In any case, they all had one thing in common in smoking practices: they mostly tried to remove negative forces from their environment. This key similarity can make learning about the German roots of incense burning interesting to any lover of incense. I hope that this book can be one entry in a worldwide chorus of historic incense traditions continued today.

When one looks at European history, one recognizes that many of the presented smoking plants were generally smoked in the European region, such as marigold or fennel, which grow in Germany but have their origins in the Mediterranean region. Certainly, some European emigrants brought their smoking herbs with them to other regions because smoking incense was something special for their ancestors; it simply belonged to their everyday life. It served as their protection, and the security they gained through it was important.

I have intentionally omitted frankincense and some other herbs, woods, and resins in my book. The reason for this is that their importation may cause harm to the vegetation of their countries of origin, such as frankincense trees, which are threatened with extinction.

Please also note that incenses follow a mental path. They do not cure diseases and certainly not depression caused by illness. Incense helps us find peace or visualize in our minds the problems we want to solve. And now I wish you inspiration and hope that you gain firsthand experience in the wonderful science of incense made from plant materials.

—Katja Peters

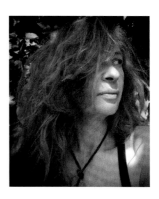

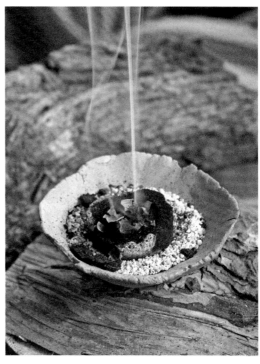

WHY DO WE BURN INCENSE?

The burning of incense made from plants is probably as old as humankind and was highly valued by our ancestors. It is assumed that Stone Age people gained experience with fragrant woods and berries around the fire. Since they could not explain at that time how this beautiful fragrance was created, they attributed magical powers to it and believed that the plant's spirit had been awakened to life.

Our ancestors burned incense to ward off weather disasters or curses from home and hearth. They believed in witches, demons, spirits, and the evil eye, all of which wanted to do them harm, such as bewitching their cattle or bringing death into the house.

As well, in some regions, pigeon lofts were smoked out with anise, fennel, and coriander, to ensure that the pigeons stayed and did not fly away. Shepherds in the Wetterau (a fertile area in the West German state of Hesse) burned cotton grass, in the belief that the smoke would protect their sheep against magic spells. The burning of incense was also used to perfume one's house and clothes with a lovely scent, to disinfect rooms, and to smoke out deadly diseases. Even coffee beans were burned for this purpose. Propolis mixed with resins was used to combat sore throat.

Small, open pans were usually used for this purpose, but special smoking pans were also employed. From today's point of view, this practice made perfect sense, because our ancestors usually selected only plants that had antibiotic or disinfectant properties and, of course, plants that warded off evil, such as rue for example. I would like to offer two examples from the former East Prussia.

The plague raged there from 1709 to 1711 and depopulated the country. It was ordered that the chambers and clothes of the deceased people be treated with smoke produced by burning amber, incense, or myrrh and juniper berries.

Source: Wilhelm Sahm, A History of the Plague in East Prussia (1905), 145

Then there is the life story of Fanny Lewald, who was born in Königsberg in 1811. In her book she tells how, while "hunger typhus" was raging, rooms were fumigated with vinegar and carnations in an incense pan in order to disinfect them, so to speak, to drive out the demon of disease. Instead of carnations, I think that she actually meant cloves, since the German word Nelke means both carnation and clove. Cloves have an antibacterial effect and exude a strong odor that, according to the belief of the time, neutralized bad smells.

Today we know that one of the primary effects of incense is to activate our senses. We all know that one associates certain smells with positive or negative feelings. Scents that we receive positively have a calming effect on us. They have a warming and protective effect on the mind and soul. This is what makes a good incense.

Also, nowadays we burn incense to achieve harmony with nature, from which we have unfortunately become very distant, or just to achieve mental peace. This is because we live in a stressful and fast-paced time and more and more people seek inner peace, which can be achieved through such practices.

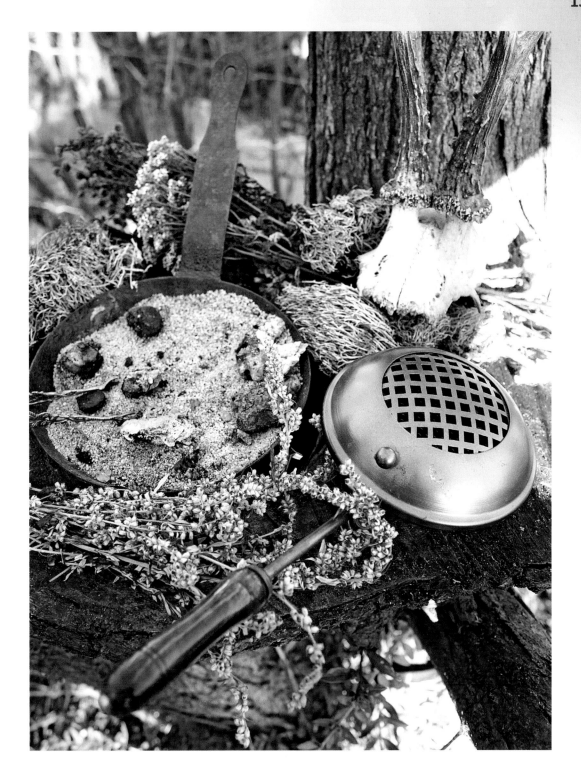

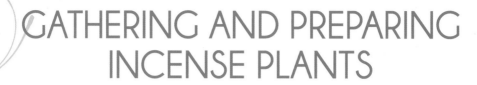

GATHERING AND PREPARING INCENSE PLANTS

The gathering of plants usually takes place from spring until the late summer, when the plants are in full bloom. In order to do justice to the endangered plant and insect world, we should plant incense herbs in our own garden or on the balcony. Personally, I grow both plants that benefit the insects and incense herbs for myself in my natural garden. So, I have herbs and the insects too. If you are unable to do this, remember the 1:10 collection rule.

This means that if you find about ten herbs growing wild in nature, take just one of them home with you. For our incense work through the fall until the following spring, we actually don't need many herbs; usually one plant per species will do. We must definitely watch out

for protected herbs, because harvesting them is restricted and in some cases forbidden! Out of respect for the natural world, I do not grow protected herbs.

The herbs that grow next to roads and fields should also not be harvested, because they have probably been contaminated by exhaust fumes and pesticides and therefore will do us more harm than good. For those who wish to purchase their incense herbs in Germany, I recommend Kräuterhaus Lindig in Munich. It has been in business since 1887 and has what I consider to be the highest-quality incense materials.

Gathering herbs should be done with dignity and respect for nature; ultimately, we are re-

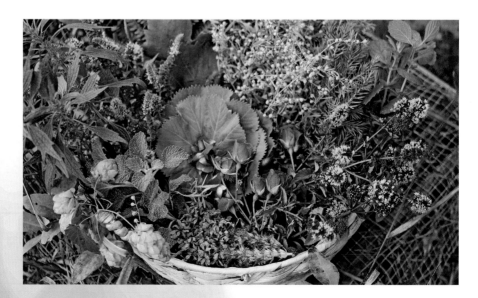

A basket filled with various herbs.

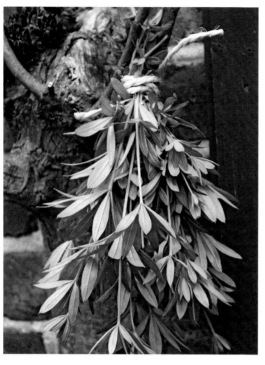
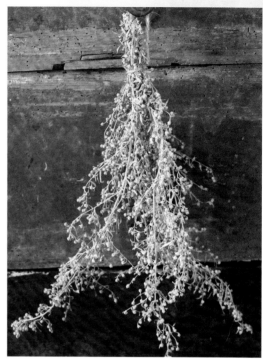

moving something that is very important to it. Therefore we should always leave something as a sign of gratitude where we have harvested herbs. Personally, I usually take oat flakes or some dried tobacco, which I lay down in small quantities where I have harvested. It is a matter of opinion whether a knife, scissors, or a ceramic blade should be used to remove the herbs. It is said that metal is not good for the herbs, since it "stresses" the plants, causing them to lose some of the good qualities that we of course need for preparing incense.

After you have harvested your herbs, they should be transported in a basket or a bag made of paper or cloth. If placed in plastic containers or bags, the herbs quickly wilt and also become mushy. If no suitable container is on hand, it would be best if you bundle the herbs and carry them home in your hand.

Most incense herbs are cut off halfway up the stalk. You should choose the most-vigorous plants—that is, the ones that have abundant flowers and leaves. Cut off the plant at the halfway point and carefully place it in your basket, taking care that nothing breaks off unnecessarily. We must always keep in mind that the plant is a living being and sacrifices its existence for us.

If you want to collect your incense herbs yourself, please make sure that you do this on dry days, because otherwise parts of the plant soon begin to mold.

Once you have gathered your herbs, proceed as you would with medicinal herbs. Hang long-stemmed herbs upside down in an airy but not sunny place. If they get too much sun during the drying process, their colors will fade and they will become very brittle. As a result, they also lose their good qualities, which we appreciate and want to use. They can safely be hung in dark spaces.

If you have just started drying herbs, you should write down exactly which plant you are drying so that you can recognize it later. Sometimes different plants look remarkably similar after they have dried. You can also hang small name tags on the plants. I lay out leaves or smaller flowers on untreated cardboard boxes that I bought especially for them, or on sandwich paper. I don't throw these papers in the trash afterward but use them again and again until they are dirty.

The parts of the plant should not touch or lie on top of each other; otherwise they may begin to mold or black-brown spots may appear. The flowers and leaves must be turned over from time to time so that they do not stick to the base.

I always place a linen cloth over the plant parts, which keeps dust from collecting and preserves their color. Especially with colorful flowers such as the cornflower with its intense blue flower color, this is a must.

Dried flowers with intense flower colors must also always be stored in the dark; otherwise they will fade.

Woods, roots, and bark are best dried on cardboard. They take a very long time to dry completely. If you have a woodstove, you can dry these incense materials on it. This speeds up the process greatly. I store wood and bark in smaller jute bags. They are good for air circulation, in case the wood still contains some residual moisture.

Tree resins take a very long time to dry. Good resin should have rested one to two years, because

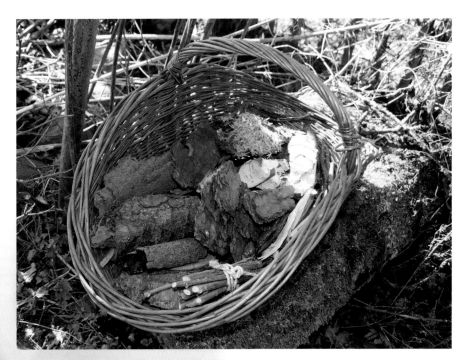

Various incense woods.

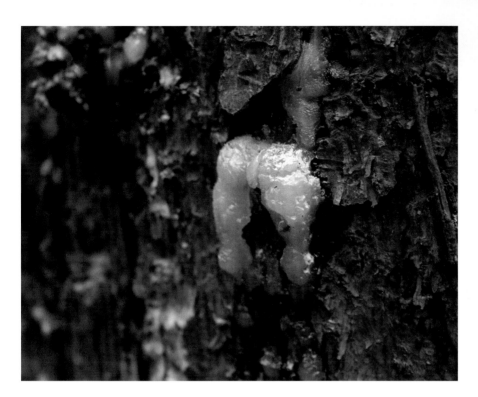

only then does it exude its proper fragrance and show its full effect. Unfortunately, resins have the property of incorporating everything when they flow down coniferous trees. This includes needles, bark, and also insects.

One only has to think of amber, which is known for revealing small fossils of insects.

Therefore, we should clean resins before using them for incense. When collecting resins, we must always be careful to remember that conifers close their wounds with the resin. Therefore, we should not scrape off any resin but should take only what runs down the wound and can be quite easily removed from the bark of the tree without causing further damage to it.

Fresh resin is very sticky. Therefore, it should be transported in a container with a lid that will not be needed again. I dry clean resin in preserving jars. I just put it in there and put the glass lid on the jar. Every once in a while, I shake the jar, and when the resin pieces no longer stick to the jar and come off, I take them out and break everything into small pieces, put them back in the jar, and then let them sit for one to two years.

Then pick out small, beautiful containers. They should be ceramic, glass, or wood. If there is not enough space to store all the containers, you can also use small paper bags.

Well-dried herbs must be flexible and "rustle" when you touch them, and they must also re-

tain their color. This is how you can tell if the herbs are done drying. Your whole dried incense plants and roots are then chopped. I always chop the whole plant, including blossoms, leaves, and stem, because we should approach this with gratitude too, to ensure that there is no waste. And if something is left over, I return it to nature. To chop it up, I take a pair of ceramic scissors and cut everything to about the size you'd find in loose herbal teas, so it's not too fine. It should be nice and crumbly, so that the dried plant parts can be easily portioned with two fingers.

Individual flowers and leaves can be placed in the storage containers whole. If you need them for an incense, just pluck or crumble the amount that you need.

Now put them in your containers and write a little note with the name of the plant. I always put the note in the container; then there are no glue residues. If you want to prepare incense mixtures, mix the selected incense ingredients 2:1, whereby the resin is always the smallest part, because it has a very strong odor when burned and would otherwise overwhelm the other incense ingredients. The resin can also be omitted, in which case the ingredients are mixed 1:1, or in equal parts.

There is no need to chop entire pieces of wood. When needed, some can be scraped off and then cut into smaller pieces. I change leaves and flowers every two years. Resins and woods I store permanently. Everything should be kept in a dark place; for example, in a cupboard or in a dark corner of the room. That is it. Now your herbs are ready to be turned into incense.

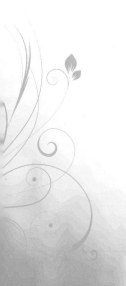

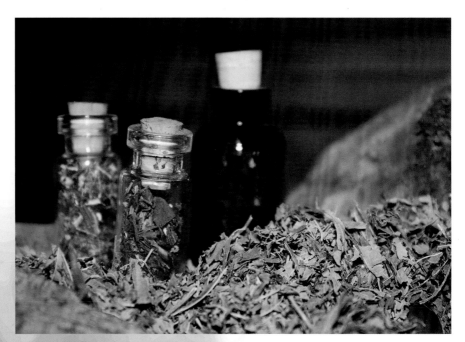

Glass vessels filled with dried herbs.

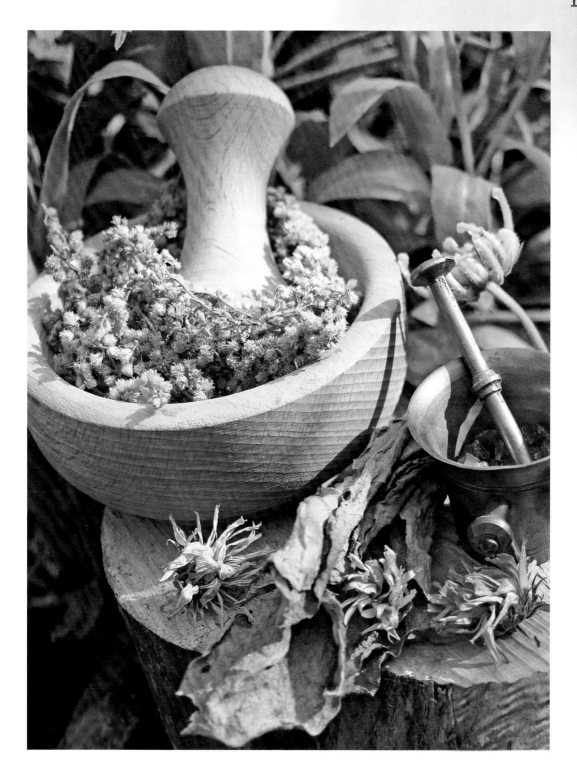

CLEANING RESINS

Coniferous resins were especially important to our ancestors. For this reason, spruce resin is also called forest incense. To get resins clean, we now have many possibilities. Unfortunately it is a very messy and sticky business. That is why the materials used should be old or specially designed for resin cleaning.

You will need a stone, a saucepan, or an empty and cleaned tin can; a stocking made of real wool (alternatively, fine-meshed gauze); a ladle; string; gloves; and a bowl. The gloves are very important because the resin can get very hot and burn the skin if you are not careful.

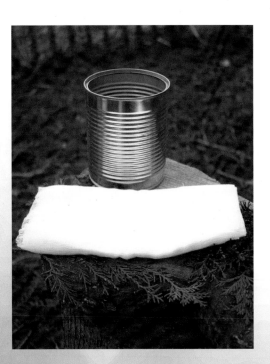

The tin can is needed in case you want to clean your resin over the campfire. Place a discarded saucepan on the burner. Now put your tree resin into the woolen sock and put a slightly larger stone into the sock. If you prefer to use gauze, make sure that the mesh is exceptionally fine. Now form it into a small bag and fill it with your resin and the stone and tie it shut. Fill the saucepan or can with water, bring to a boil, and then reduce the heat to the lowest setting. When the water has come to a boil, put your resin bag in the ladle and place it in the water. The stone acts as a weight to keep the bag submerged. After a while you will see that the hot water causes the resin to liquefy. It then rises through the sock or gauze to the surface of the water.

Now fill the bowl with cold water. Using the ladle, scoop out the hot water with the hot resin and pour it into the cold water in the bowl. The resin cools down immediately and becomes solid again. When you take it out, you can also form it into sticks, balls, and chunks. Afterward the pieces are laid out on parchment paper to harden. The same rule applies here: the longer a resin is stored, the more intense is its smell and its beneficial properties for the body and mind.

The resin is now left in the open for a few days to harden and then placed into jars, as I explain in the chapter "Gathering and Preparing Incense Plants." Purified spruce resin is also called burgundy resin.

When collecting resin, it is essential to ensure that it is not taken indiscriminately from the co-

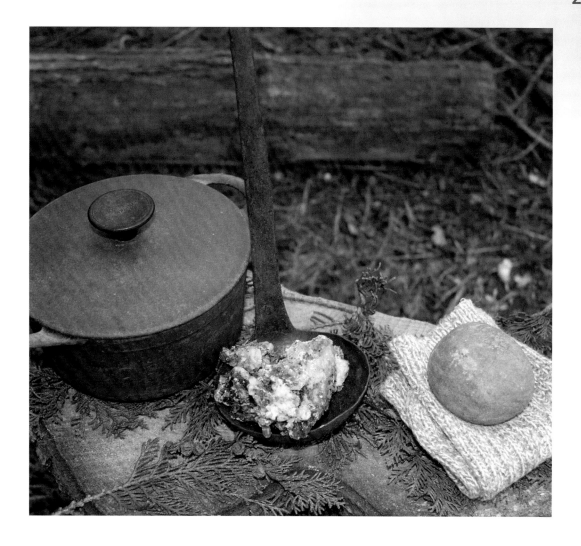

nifers. It is vital to the coniferous tree for sealing wounds. If we were to take it from there, we would automatically reopen the wound.

The resin performs a function similar to that of a scab on a wound. That's why we should keep an eye out for fallen trees or look for trees with resin dripping directly from the resin cap. This can be collected with a clear conscience. Sometimes we are also lucky to find a place where the dripping resin has collected right at the base of the coniferous tree or on the forest floor around the trunk.

I have planted a Scots pine and spruces in my natural garden especially for the purpose of resin extraction. If there is insufficient space in your garden, conifers can also be cultivated in a large tub.

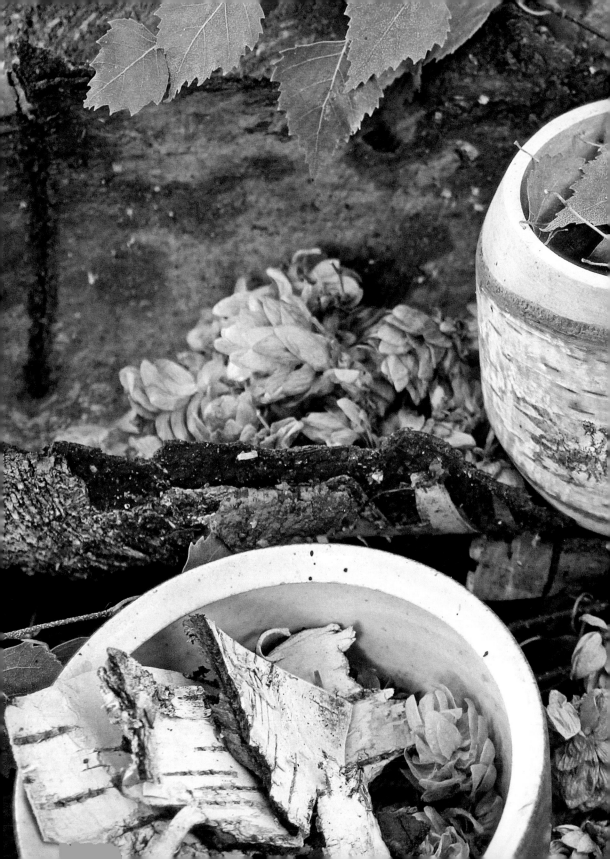

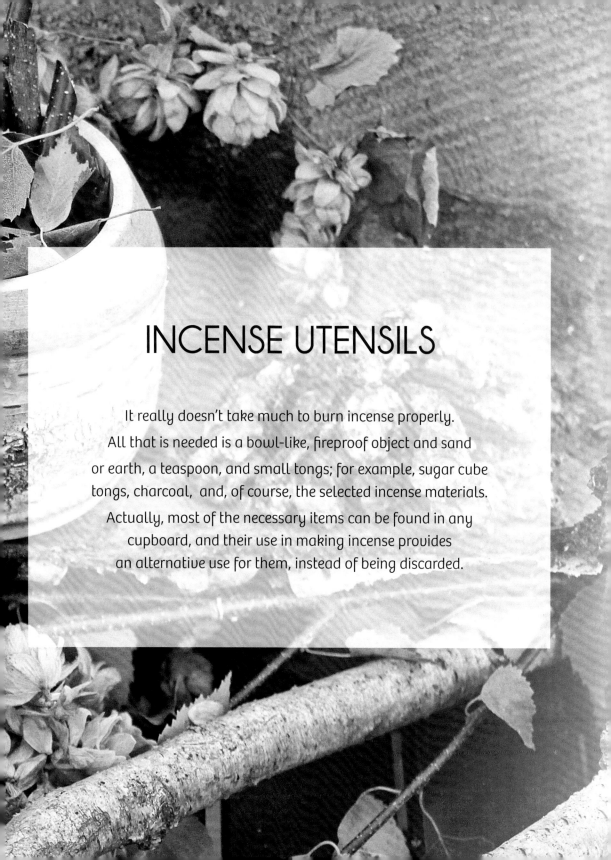

INCENSE UTENSILS

It really doesn't take much to burn incense properly.
All that is needed is a bowl-like, fireproof object and sand
or earth, a teaspoon, and small tongs; for example, sugar cube
tongs, charcoal, and, of course, the selected incense materials.

Actually, most of the necessary items can be found in any
cupboard, and their use in making incense provides
an alternative use for them, instead of being discarded.

INCENSE CONTAINERS

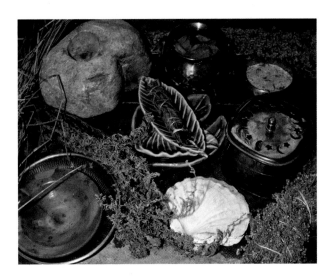

I like to use seashells, fieldstones with a large depression, small clay pots, and small antique iron pans for burning incense. If you want something special, you should look on the internet; there is much from this area on offer. The safest and most authentic are incense pans with lids. They are available in different sizes and designs.

INCENSE SAND

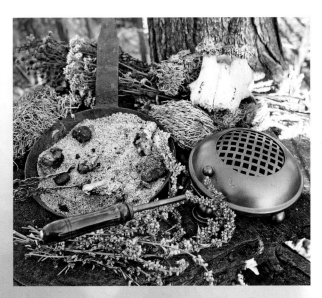

Many people use craft sand, but soil taken from nature can also be used. It must be well screened and dried prior to use.

TONGS AND SPOONS

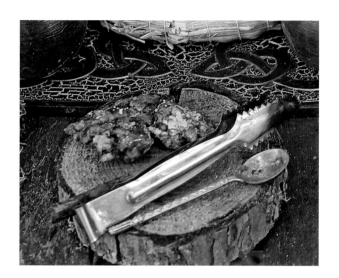

There are really nice tongs for sugar cubes and loose sugar spoons, which are usually a little wider. The tongs are there to light your incense charcoal. I use the spoon when I want to extinguish the incense, by sprinkling some earth or sand over it.

INCENSE CHARCOAL

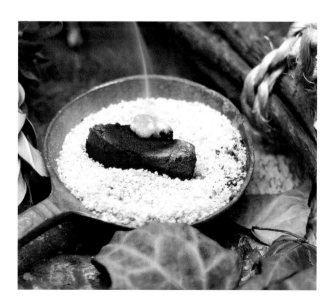

As described on page 26, you can make your own incense charcoal with a tinder fungus. As well, if you have a woodstove in the house, untreated charcoal can be taken from it. There are also incense charcoal tablets, which can be bought locally or on the internet. The only drawback is that one never knows how they were made, which of course is important for us since we burn incense in the house. Such an incense for our senses should be made as naturally as possible.

NATURAL INCENSE CHARCOAL

Incense charcoal can be made using a tinder fungus. In the past it was grasped with tongs and held inverted in the stove for a few minutes, and when it started to glow a little bit, the incense material, preferably tree resin, such as that from the Swiss stone pine or spruce, was rubbed on the smooth undersurface, which was facing upward. This method was used in Alpine regions to smoke out rooms during wintertime.

Nowadays, charcoal tablets are imported from far away, and we have no idea if the way they are produced harms the environment or if they contain harmful additives. When burning incense, we should always make sure that all the incense, along with the charcoal, is free from harmful substances, because we automatically inhale these when we burn incense.

The tinder fungus, a native tree fungus, is ideally suited for this purpose. From it comes the saying "It burns like tinder." This mushroom smolders for a very long time without spraying sparks. In the Middle Ages, smoldering tinder fungi were carried by travelers to enable them to make a fire while on the journey.

For this purpose, the tinder fungus was specially treated. Tinder fungus is found mostly on dead trees, such as beech or birch. It can be easily separated from the wood, except for older specimens. They sit very tightly on the wood, but if you strike the large underside of the fungus with the palm of your hand, it can be dislodged and removed. For our incense charcoal, we should look only for impeccable tinder fungi. This can be determined by examining the underside of the fungus.

It must not be perforated or show any traces of feeding; such fungi usually contain insects. Taking such fungi would be equivalent to taking the insects' homes and destroying them.

One also has to look for small holes on the top. The tinder fungus must look flawless all around. You can take such a specimen home with you. One fungus is enough.

For our natural incense charcoal, we must tackle the inside of this fungus, the so-called trama. I use the word "tackle," because it is a very hard fungus and a saw can easily slip off. Therefore one must use caution and preferably wear sturdy gloves.

The fungus must first be cut in two. When you have done this, you will see a brown crumbly substance, the trama, under the tubes and crust. This substance is the tinder, our natural incense charcoal.

It is removed from the fungus and cut into pieces. Now you can take a piece of tinder with a small pair of tongs and light it. The fastest and easiest way is with a burning candle.

After a while you will see the piece of tinder start to glow. Blow on it repeatedly, because this causes the embers to ignite more quickly.

The glowing tinder can now be placed on the bottom of your incense burner, and your incense can be placed on the embers with a small spoon or tongs. The remaining tinder can be stored can be stored in small wooden boxes.

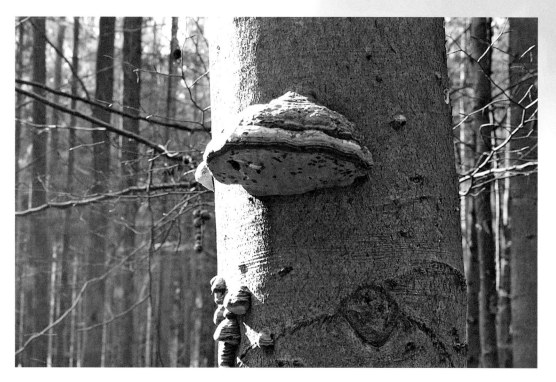

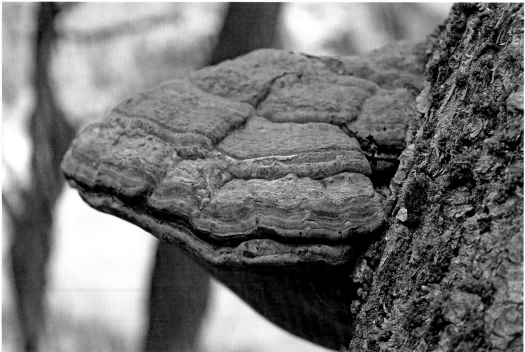

Two examples of tinder fungi.

THE PROPER WAY TO BURN INCENSE

Nowadays there are so many ways to burn incense that there is something for every taste. I myself prefer to do it rustically, the way it was done in earlier times. All I need is a container, charcoal, tongs, and my incense material. When we burn incense made from plant parts, the object is to release the plant spirit from its matter, since this gives to us its very own plant power.

To burn incense as it was done in earlier times, one needs a small fireproof bowl, clean soil, tinder fungus or glowing wood charcoal, tongs, a teaspoon, and incense.

Pour the soil into your bowl and ignite the wood charcoal (or tinder fungus) until it glows, then place it in the center of the soil. It must be thoroughly glowing. If I do not have tinder fungus on hand, I often take glowing embers from my stove. Now you can begin burning your incense. Best to start with a knife tip full and test your way through the various plants. Some herbs will appeal to you, and others you will avoid. It depends on how we absorb it. When it comes to resins, the rule is "less is more."

Resin tends to produce a great deal of smoke. Therefore it is sufficient to put just a little on the embers.

You can add more as needed. Whether or not your windows should be open depends on what you are burning the incense for. If it has to do with house cleaning, several windows should be opened, so that the smoke can disperse and take all the old tales out into the open air. When it comes to your peace of mind, I recommend keeping the windows closed, so that you can burn incense and let it work its magic on your mind and body. After that, I open the windows. Burning incense out in nature, of course, is a very special experience. Through this we get closer to Mother Nature and become more open to connect with her. Incense is about visualizing wishes, dreams, and also solutions to problems in the mind's eye to obtain an answer, but also just to get peace and balance. Of course, we can also perform whole ceremonies or rituals. The best way to do this is to go out into nature so that we can ground ourselves.

As you can see, it is really not difficult, and after some time everyone will develop his or her own style of burning incense.

Incense plants with powerful properties usually have a very intense scent.

In the past, stronger-smelling herbs were said to have certain abilities. It was believed that the scent and the plant spirit gave help, protection, and security.

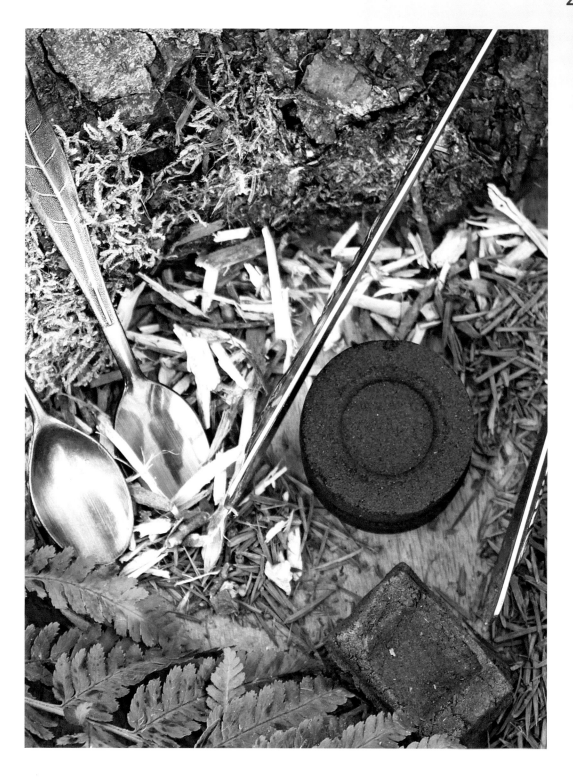

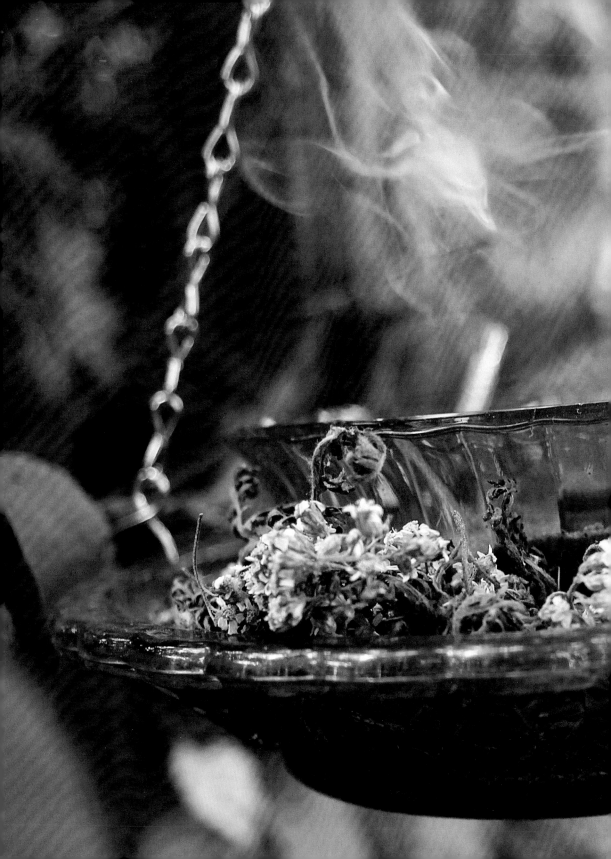

BURNING INCENSE AT DIFFERENT TIMES OF YEAR

The different seasons used to be very important to people. Seasonal festivities were celebrated, betrothals were made, and thanks were given for the harvest, and of course incense was burned on these occasions. Plant-based incense was used for the most part, since it fit into these seasons or had a high value in folk belief, because people then believed that it provided protection for the home, farm, and fields or helped the residents remain healthy until the next year.

These incenses were important at that time because people used to regard everything as "animate." If, for example, one was at home at night with no electricity or car noise, no water pipes, sitting in a wooden house with pine shavings on the floor, one was surrounded by spirits and demons. One could hear the wood creaking, mice running across the attic, or the wind making eerie noises. These incenses gave people support and security.

We should also note that the earlier annual-cycle festivals were determined by the moon and the sun. The calendar came only much later.

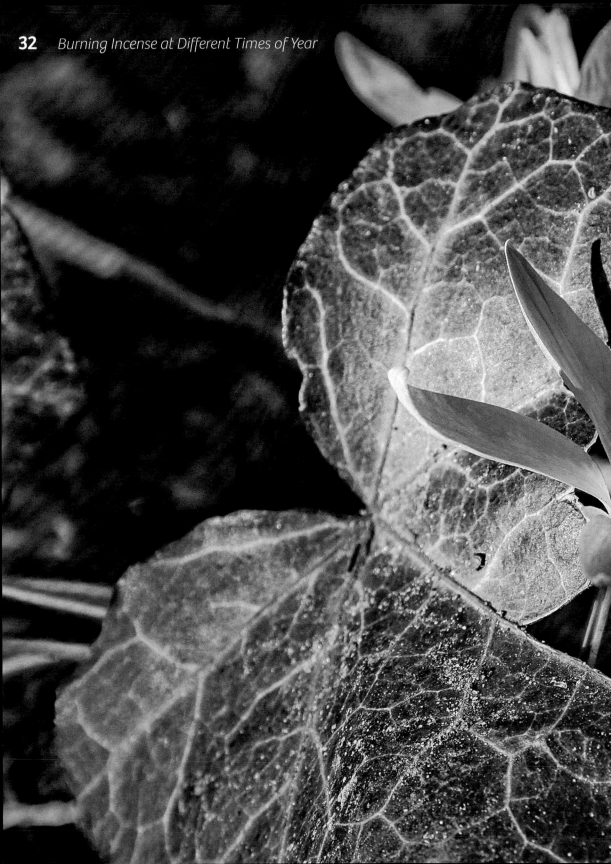

The Spring Equinox

This beautiful seasonal festival is celebrated between March 20 and 22 and marks the beginning of spring. It honors the return of longer days and the sun. In the past, marriages were performed and fields were cultivated at this time, because the returning light also brings back the fertility of nature, which was especially important for survival at that time. The spring equinox is dominated by the color yellow, and that is why yellow spring flowers, such as the cowslip, are regarded as the messengers of light. These spring flowers were of course also used to decorate the house and yard.

An incense at this time of year should be made of larch resin, coltsfoot, birch bark, woodruff, ground ivy, and blossoms from the cowslip. All incense substances must be well dried beforehand. Then they are crushed and mixed in equal parts, with the exception of the larch resin. I recommend that to make this incense you use three parts of the plant mixture and one part larch resin.

With this incense we celebrate the returning sun, which is very important to us humans, even nowadays. It scares away the gray winter, the cold, and the bleakness. The garden begins to sprout, and soon the gathering of herbs will begin again. We go out into nature more often, and our feelings improve from day to day. The sun means life.

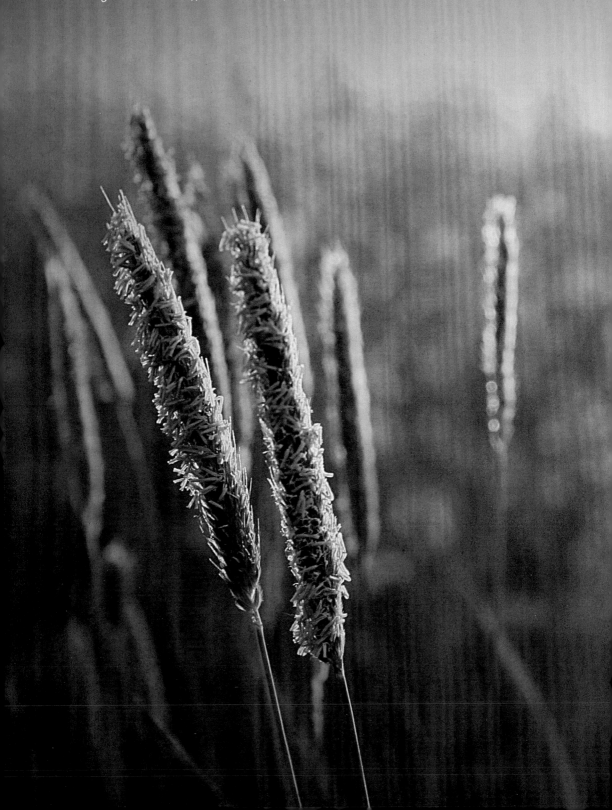

The Summer Solstice

Everyone has heard or read about this seasonal festival. It is the beginning of summer and is celebrated during the period from June 21 to 23. By then the sun has reached its highest point, and unfortunately from that day onward, the days again begin to get shorter. There are many folk beliefs and rites entwined with this festival. The St. John's herbs come from this period. These include not only St. John's wort, but also all the healing herbs that grow at this time of year. They have great healing power and the ability to ward off all evil, according to folk belief.

These St. John's herbs were especially important. They were attributed with purifying and cleansing properties. They were also regarded as magical. It was believed that the old should go in order to let the new arise. Solstice bundles were also tied at this time. These bundles consisted of various St. John's herbs, which were tied and hung upside down to dry. When needed—to ward off bad weather or illness—the respective herb was then taken from the bundle and burned as incense or drunk as a tea.

St. John's herbs definitely include St. John's wort, oregano, mugwort, oak leaves, clover (red and white), hare leaf, lady's mantle, mint, nettle, and rosehip branches, but also any other plant that blooms at this time of year and is not poisonous. These herbs can be mixed to make a summer solstice incense. It should always include three, seven, or nine different herbs—which our ancestors believed were magic numbers.

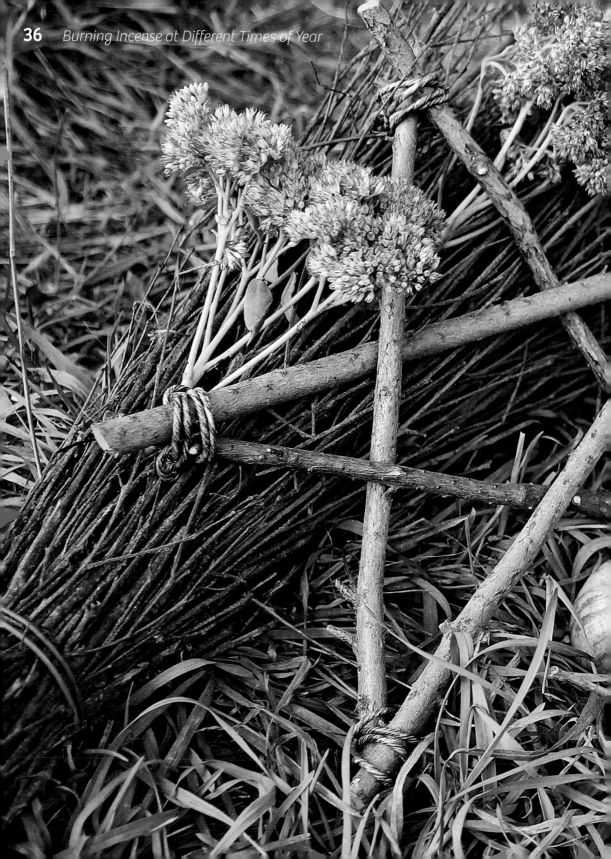

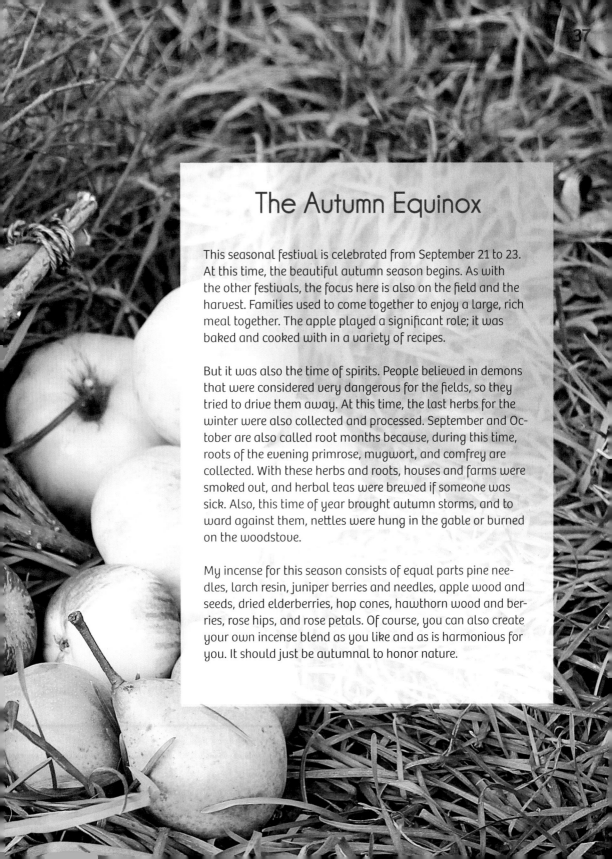

The Autumn Equinox

This seasonal festival is celebrated from September 21 to 23. At this time, the beautiful autumn season begins. As with the other festivals, the focus here is also on the field and the harvest. Families used to come together to enjoy a large, rich meal together. The apple played a significant role; it was baked and cooked with in a variety of recipes.

But it was also the time of spirits. People believed in demons that were considered very dangerous for the fields, so they tried to drive them away. At this time, the last herbs for the winter were also collected and processed. September and October are also called root months because, during this time, roots of the evening primrose, mugwort, and comfrey are collected. With these herbs and roots, houses and farms were smoked out, and herbal teas were brewed if someone was sick. Also, this time of year brought autumn storms, and to ward against them, nettles were hung in the gable or burned on the woodstove.

My incense for this season consists of equal parts pine needles, larch resin, juniper berries and needles, apple wood and seeds, dried elderberries, hop cones, hawthorn wood and berries, rose hips, and rose petals. Of course, you can also create your own incense blend as you like and as is harmonious for you. It should just be autumnal to honor nature.

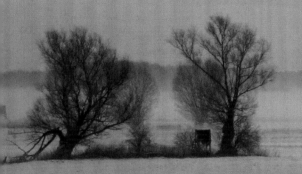

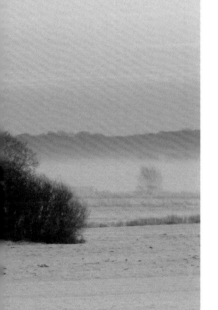

The Winter Solstice

The winter solstice marks the beginning of winter and is celebrated between December 21 and 22. From that time onward, the days become longer again. The return of the sun is now expected and honored by large celebrations. Families celebrate with games and big meals. The fire was of course part of the celebration.

The houses were cleaned and polished and there was much baking—in the shape of animals and suns. On hills, large wheels were wrapped with straw, set on fire, and rolled down burning. They embodied the returning sun.

Of course, on these cold evenings there was also much burning of incense made from plants. Suitable plants at this time are mugwort, ash, toadstools, mistletoe, elderflowers, sloe, spruce resin, and juniper berries or wood.

The burning of incense always began in the cattle shed because cattle were the most-valuable possessions that people had at that time. After that, the house was smoked out, not forgetting the corners. A lot of mugwort was burned because it was believed to keep everything negative away from the house and property. You can also make a special incense mixture from different plant parts for the winter solstice.

The Twelve Nights

This period has various names in Germany, such as *Rauhnächte* or *die Zwölften*, the spelling depending on from which region one comes. In old books one often reads about *Rauchnächten* (literally "incense-burning nights"), which sounds very consistent to me, since the burning of incense is related to smoke (*Rauch*) and there is much burning of incense on these nights.

There are so many customs for these incense-burning nights that they would fill several books. The incense-burning nights are the famous "Twelve Nights." The custom differs from region to region, including the number of nights: sometimes there are only three. In any case, a lot of incense was burned during this time in order to receive the maximum blessings and protection. On those nights the main Germanic god, Wotan, also known as Odin, flew through the air with his wild army and thus caused much noise and din. It is also called the *Wilde Jagd* (the Ferocious Pursuit). I think we can compare it today with the winter storms that occurred more often at that time, as a metaphor for the winter storm. For these twelve nights the people made from a cross from a hazel switch and an elder branch to keep the Ferocious Pursuit away.

On December 25, frankincense, twigs of blackthorn, and the herbs consecrated for Easter were burned in an incense burner.

I think that before Christianity became widespread, it was certainly coniferous resin that was burned instead of frankincense.

The process began in the cattle sheds, and after that the incense pan was carried through the house, room by room. For those who could afford it, the ceremony was carried out by the local priest; otherwise it was done by the householder himself.

When the incense burning was completed, they went to bed, but before doing so they were supposed to symbolically make a cross on the floor with the left foot, so that no witch or nightmare could creep up to the bed.

These "incense-burning nights" were nature at a standstill, for it was not until twelve nights after the winter solstice that a change, the longer days caused by the returning sun, became apparent. These twelve nights are supposed to compensate for the missing days in the lunar year. The lunar year has 354 days, and a solar year 365–366 days. Our ancestors lived according to the lunar year.

The burning of incense was very popular at this time of year. Incense was burned using the charcoal from the wood burned on Holy Saturday. If incense was burned throughout the house and cattle shed, nothing was allowed to be dropped. Mostly people used speick root (Valeriana celtica—a kind of Valerian) and frankincense/spruce resin.

In addition, prayers were said to drive away witches and evil spirits. Nowadays an incense made from mugwort, wormwood, elder wood, sloe wood, mistletoe, spruce resin, and juniper is burned.

It is a beautiful time for inner contemplation and to reflect with a cup of herbal tea and incense on how one would like to start the new year. This is the time for small board games, Tarot, oracle, and also rituals. Simply come to rest, bring to an end the everyday life of the old year, say goodbye to the old year, and welcome the new.

SPECIAL INCENSES USED BY OUR ANCESTORS

Some incense practices are very special and have been handed down to the present time. Our ancestors were very inventive and did not just create incense from plants and resins, but also with sweepings from all four corners of the room. They believed that in this way everything negative was swept out and burned.

The soles from shoes, fingernails, hair, and everything imaginable was also burned, in order to obtain protection against any evil forces. This is usually not written about, because it does not fit at all into our time.

NINE WOODS

Nine woods was always used as a defensive spell, as incense, an amulet, or a talisman, or also in the form of a bath. Roma and Sinti carried nine woods in a small linen pouch around the hips or neck, for protection against wasting diseases such as cancer. If one wants to make such an amulet, then it must include hazel.

Nine woods is a folk belief that has its roots in the magic number 9. It was believed that nine different woods possessed great power. Which wood was taken from which tree or shrub depended on what it was needed for.

In earlier times, people upon whom a negative spell had been cast were treated with smoke produced by burning nine kinds of wood. It was also called a "need-fire." "Nine woods" was also used to protect one's house and belongings.

For this purpose, the woods were stuck into the ground around the yard. The woods were also hung in the cattle sheds, to prevent intruders from getting in. A combination of cherry, plum, pear, apple, fir, pine, birch, linden, and willow wood was used to counter spells placed on livestock. Apart from that, the tree species were not allowed to end in "tree."

Nine woods—specifically apple, pear, lilac, elder, gooseberry, currant, hornbeam, poplar, and wild rose—was also used to treat headache. If children developed a rash, they were given a nine-woods bath using woods from fruit trees, dried thyme, and reeds. Or the woods were simply carried in a trouser pocket for protection against witches. Woods from the aspen, oak, pine, beech, linden, rowan, spruce, fir, and birch trees were used for this purpose.

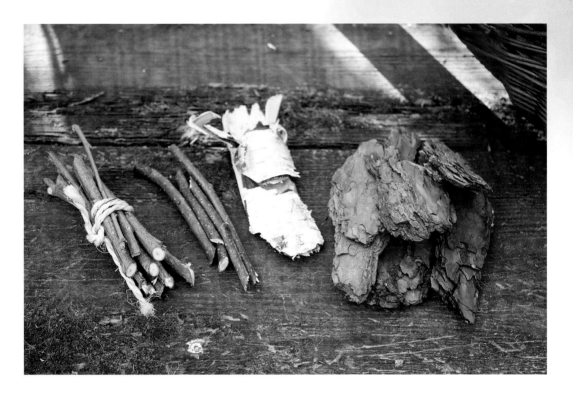

The nine woods had to be gathered quietly in the forest and could not be cut from living bushes or trees. Instead, the wood that was collected was found lying on the ground. The various types included the spruce, fir, larch, Scots pine, yew, stone pine, mountain pine, juniper, sade tree (stink juniper), oak, beech, linden, maple, birch, hazel, aspen, and rowan. Generally these woods were considered to be very effective for warding off evil. They were often used as incense.

In addition, there is also the belief in nine herbs. This custom dates back to pagan times and was continued after the arrival of Christianity. Here, nine different herbs play a role, and they are sorted differently from region to region.

The origin of this folk belief can be seen in the Germanic peoples because it is attributed to the nine healing goddesses. They were invoked in those days and asked for cures. Therefore, the nine woods also belongs to the plant sacrifices. One "sacrificed" plant parts after a certain ritual, in order to receive healing from the healing goddesses. Mostly these herbs were collected after a specific ritual. The most important of these herbs were elecampane, valerian, mugwort, oregano, verbena, oats, St. John's wort, tansy, and yarrow. They were bundled or crushed and dried and burned as incense against all kinds of misfortune.

In the Masurian region, on St. John's Eve cows were given nine herbs with flour and salt to protect them against spells and to ensure that they gave plenty of good milk.

BELIEF IN MALEFICENCE

Maleficent powder was the universal powder used by our ancestors. It was made from herbs and was believed to have apotropaic properties, providing protection against evil or bad luck. According to their beliefs, it helped against everything. It was, so to speak, their balm for the soul, which had a calming effect and took away all harmful spells. Since our ancestors were very superstitious, they saw danger that could harm everywhere, from people and animals to natural phenomena. Our ancestors even tried to protect their homes and property with maleficent powder.

The best-known plant used in the production of the famous maleficent powder was the wood avens. Its fragrant root was believed to ward off witches and drive away demons. It was dried and powdered and was the main ingredient used to make maleficent powder or maleficent incense. Its root has always been used to "drive out" evil spirits, demons, and the devil. It was also hung inside the house to ward off any harm. Powdered avens root was spread in the form of a circle. One then stepped inside the circle and was protected against negative influences. In order to treat diseases brought on by spells, the affected area was exposed to incense smoke, oiled, and then covered with a maleficent plaster. This process was repeated several times. The same treatment was used to ward off the evil eye.

Here is a list of ingredients for a maleficent powder from the eighteenth century:

MALEFICENT POWDER

Rue, rose petals (no floral leaves), St. John's wort blossoms, marjoram, juniper berries, pine resin, mugwort, hazel catkin, oak leaves, and wood avens root.

All incense substances are added in equal parts, the exception being the avens root, which formed a higher percentage of the mixture. All the incense ingredients had to be dried before mixing. The pine resin was supposed to have been stored for at least a year.

Facing page:
Wood avens root.

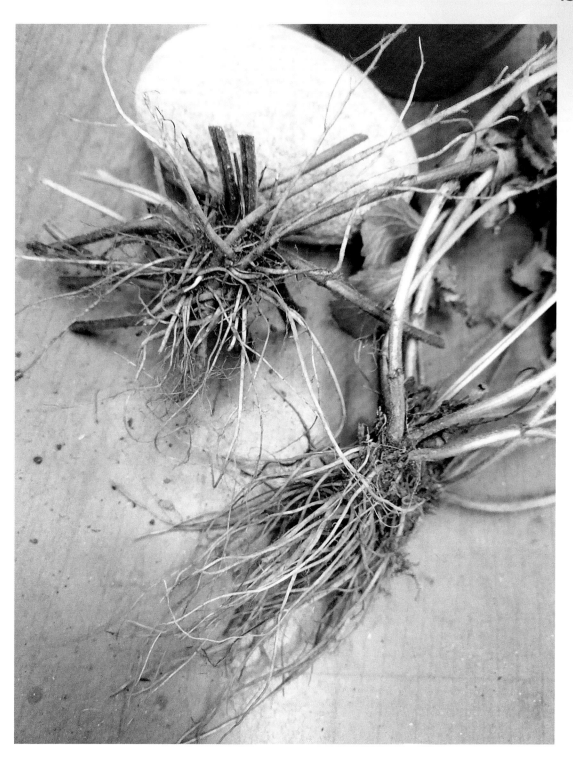

THE FLY AGARIC MUSHROOM

Incense has always been made from the fly agaric mushroom. Please note, since this is a poisonous incense ngredient (even to the touch), it is being described here for informational purposes only. Do not attempt to touch, forage, burn, or use this mushroom in any way.

This incense is used by some experts to ask questions about the future. Questions about the future sometimes torment us, because in many matters we want to know what our actions and behavior will bring us. The spirit of the fly agaric mushroom opens doors and gateways to the future. It opens our consciousness and thus enables us to look into the future. It is used by some advanced practitioners as an incense for asking questions about the future, receiving answers, and interpreting them correctly. The fly agaric mushroom shows people mystery, divine knowledge, and spiritual power.

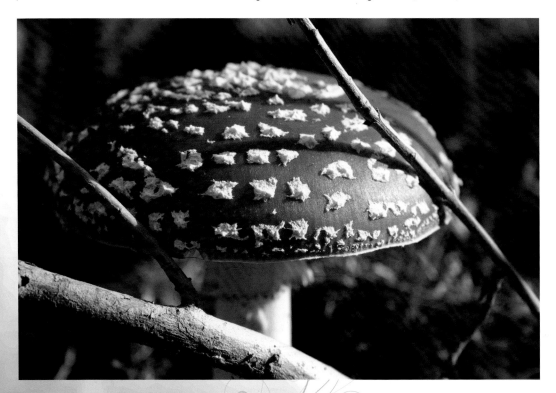

Facing page:
Fly agaric mushroom on damp soil under fir trees.

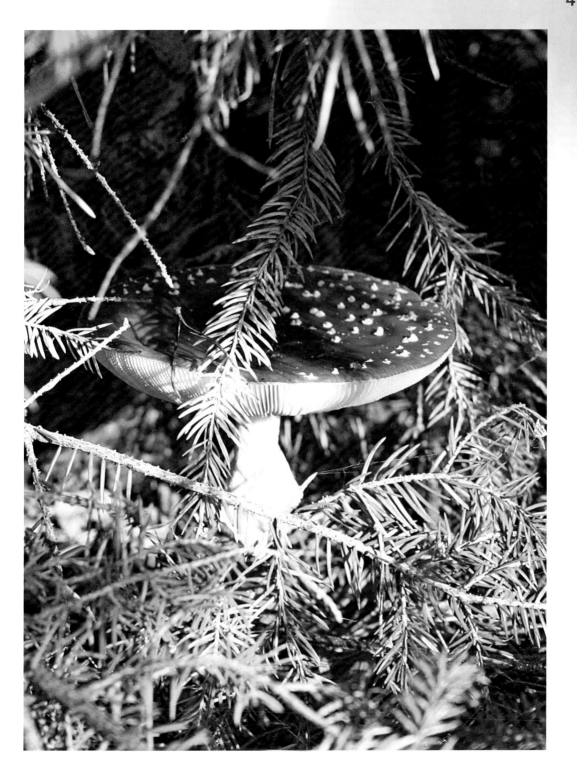

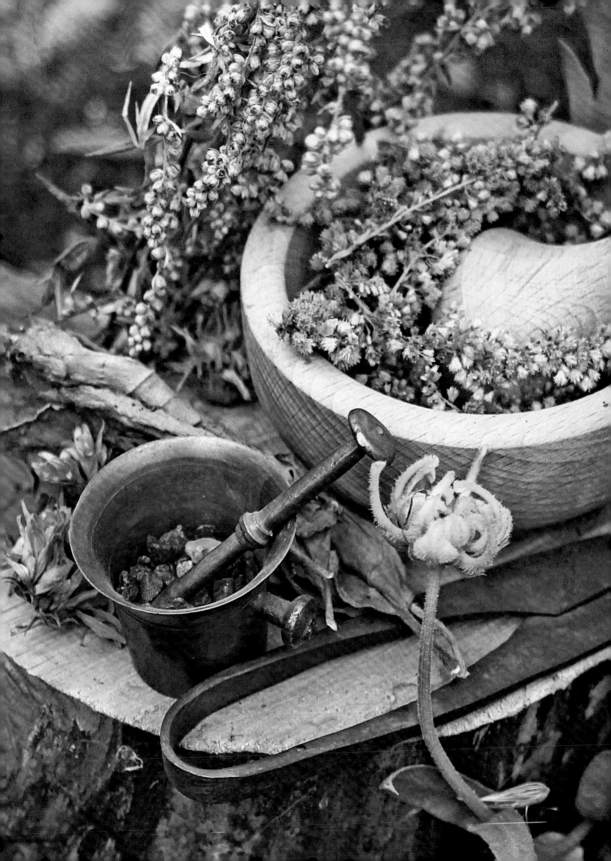

INCENSE PLANT
LEXICON

Here I will present thirty-five incense substances that had great
importance in the incense lore of our ancestors and still do even
today. I associate each plant with a message
to us incense connoisseurs.

The old incense lore is something special, because that which was
very important to our ancestors at that time, sometimes even
seeming essential for survival, has become foreign to us today.
Which is also good, because often in the past, things were burned
that nowadays would be considered repugnant, such as old shoe
soles, sweepings, or even fingernails.

Burning parts of old brooms with which one had previously
swept out a negatively charged room was also
very popular. I think that we neither want nor need
such things today.

ANGELICA

Angelica Archangelica

Back to Our Roots

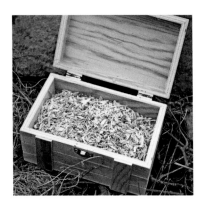

Angelica achieves its greatest protective potential against black magic. Old houses are still cleansed with it and thus regain their positive energies. Therefore, these roots are a must when one burns incense for expulsion and protection. To receive visions, the roots alone were burned.

Angelica root incense was popular in the middle of winter and during Samhain (a festival marking the end of the harvest and the beginning of winter, or the "darker half of the year"). Its plant spirit gives us warmth and protection in these seasons of transition. In those times it was also burned to fight diseases of any kind. For this purpose, the roots were burned in an incense pan, which was waved through the rooms. Angelica incense was also used against the evil eye and evil spells. The dried roots were also hung around the necks of children like a necklace to protect them.

Angelica gives us the strength to find our way back to our roots and also to generate self-confidence, which is especially important for new ventures in life.

If we want to send a wish to our ancestors, we should burn incense made from the roots of the angelica. According to ancient beliefs, they open the door to the other world. If you go to collect the roots yourself, please note that you should dry them quickly, because they are susceptible to insect damage.

Angelica roots have a very peculiar smell. Since time immemorial, angelica has been a part of every protective incense.

A mixture of angelica roots, juniper, and oregano is particularly suitable for such a protective incense.

WHERE AND WHEN TO GATHER

Angelica can be found on damp roadsides or meadows, but is more easily found in Europe than in North America and may have to be cultivated. It is collected from April to October. Seeds, roots, and even the leaves can be collected and dried.

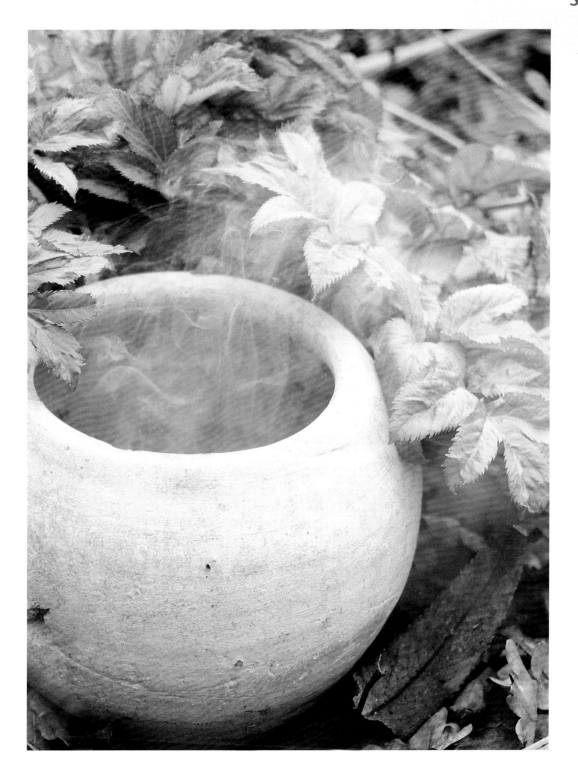

BLACK ELDER / ELDERBERRY

Sambucus Nigra

A Magical Incense

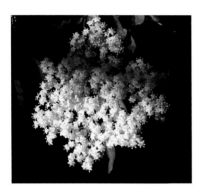

Burning incense made with elderberry has inspired humankind since time immemorial. Among the Germanic tribes, elder was the protective tree of the family. Its wood could not be used as firewood and burned, because in doing so the fire released the trapped spirits, causing misfortune to befall one. The utmost caution is therefore always called for if one makes a fire with elder.

Elderberry draws all the troubles present in a property and its inhabitants into its soil, and by burning the wood we would release this evil into our living spaces again. This custom was once firmly anchored in folk beliefs, especially among the Roma and Sinti. Using elder as firewood was taboo to them.

By burning incense with the dried blossoms, we can ask about our destiny. Their smoke creates a slightly buoyant atmosphere, which tells our spirit the right time to finish something that we may have been putting off for a long time.

It is and always has been used as a protective incense. Incense with elder heals our soul and causes us to sleep, so that we come to rest. The dried flowers are used for this purpose. To make a mentally healing and clarifying incense, the elder should be smoked pure. It is also used in incense-burning ceremonies to honor our ancestors. For this, the flowers and leaves are used.

WHERE AND WHEN TO GATHER

Elderberry often grows at the edges of forests. Its plant parts can be gathered from April until into September, while elderberry wood can be harvested the whole year round.

The wood of the elderberry can also be added to the incense. The pith, leaves, dried flowers, and dried berries can also be used. Elder mixes well with St. John's wort or fennel (or both) to produce a magical incense.

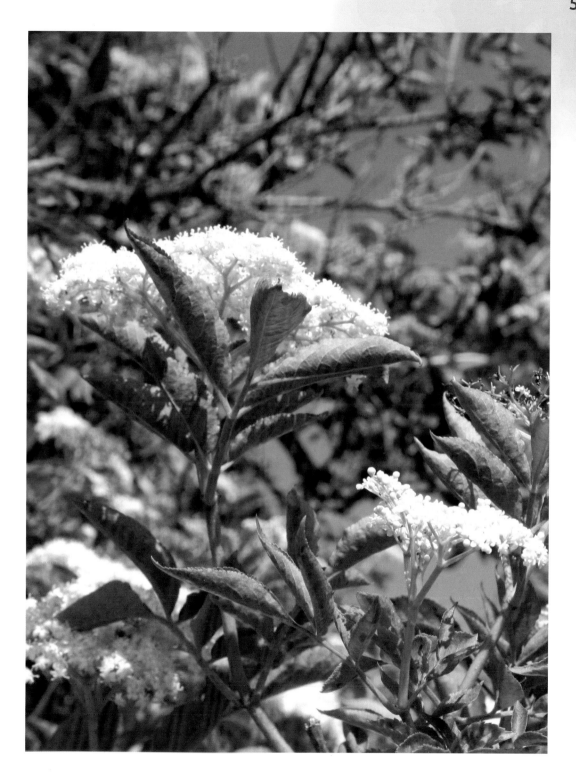

COMFREY
Symphytum Officinale
Mischief-Preventing Roots

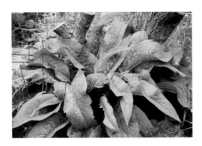

Comfrey was formerly used to smoke out sickrooms. Special smoking pans were used for this purpose. These were lidded pans with holes in the lid through which the smoke could escape.

The comfrey's roots were said to have miraculous powers, because they were capable of dispelling demons, meaning diseases.

But it is also characterized by its powerful repellent properties. In those times, and not just in the Middle Ages, people often burned this incense in large quantities to ward off everything bad: misfortune affecting the family, illnesses, witchcraft, thefts, and also the weather (e.g., lightning strikes).

In modern incense making we use the plant's flowers, leaves, and roots to remove barricades and block fears of the future. The plant spirit gently accompanies us on intentional trance journeys into our inner being. It strengthens our self-confidence and grounds us with Mother Nature.

WHERE AND WHEN TO GATHER

Comfrey likes to grow wild in meadows and on fallow land. It is present everywhere, often at the edges of fields. For an incense, you need the roots, which must be washed after they are dug up, cut into small pieces and dried very quickly. Unfortunately, they tend to mold quickly. Therefore, you need to check that there is no residual moisture after drying. For use as an incense, you can gather the roots all year round.

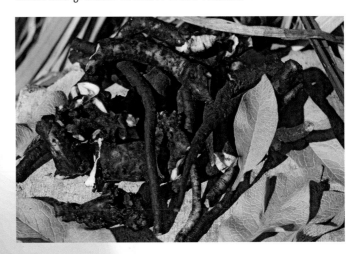

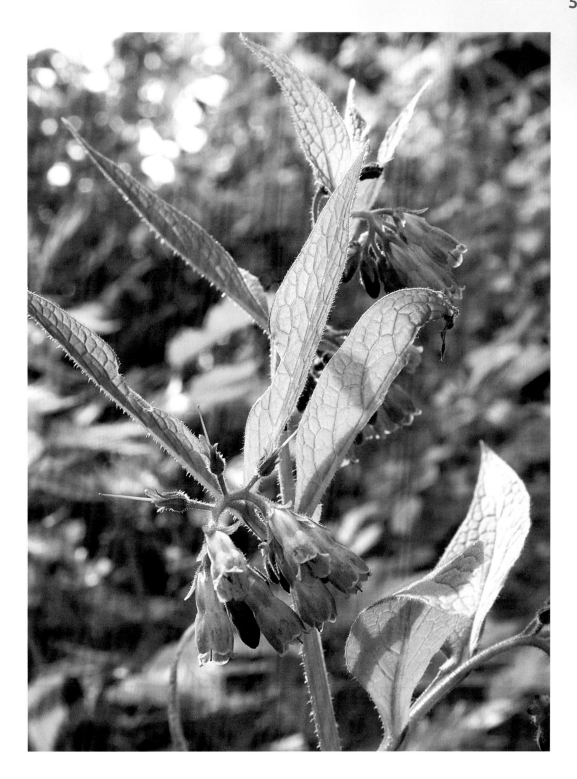

ELECAMPANE
Inula Helenium

Dispels Depressive Moods

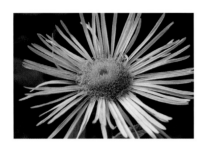

Elecampane has a long tradition in the familiar herb bundles. From this you can see how important this plant was in folklore. In the north of Germany, it had its place in the middle of the bundle instead of mullein. In case of calamity, whether from disease or bad weather, parts of this bundle were burned as incense so that nothing bad would happen. Therefore, elecampane belongs to the protective plants. In the past, its roots were also burned to ward off mosquitoes.

In incense lore, its fragrant roots were the mostly widely used part of the plant. When smoked, they have a purifying and protective effect. Our spirit is cleansed, and depressive moods are dispelled. But the roots were also burned as incense for those who were grieving.

If we have the feeling that people wish us ill, elecampane can be burned to dispel evil spells and curses.

WHERE AND WHEN TO GATHER

In some locations in North America and Europe, you can find Elecampane in wet places or having escaped from gardens. For the most part, Elecampane should be grown in the garden or purchased from herbal pharmacies on the internet.

Its collection time is late summer, early August, when it is in full bloom. If you want to collect the roots, you should wait until the flowering has passed, so that the power has flowed back into the roots.

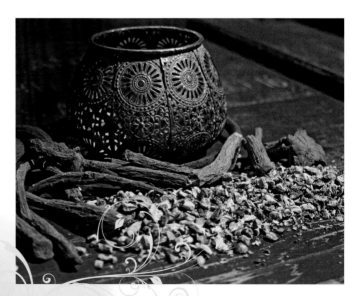

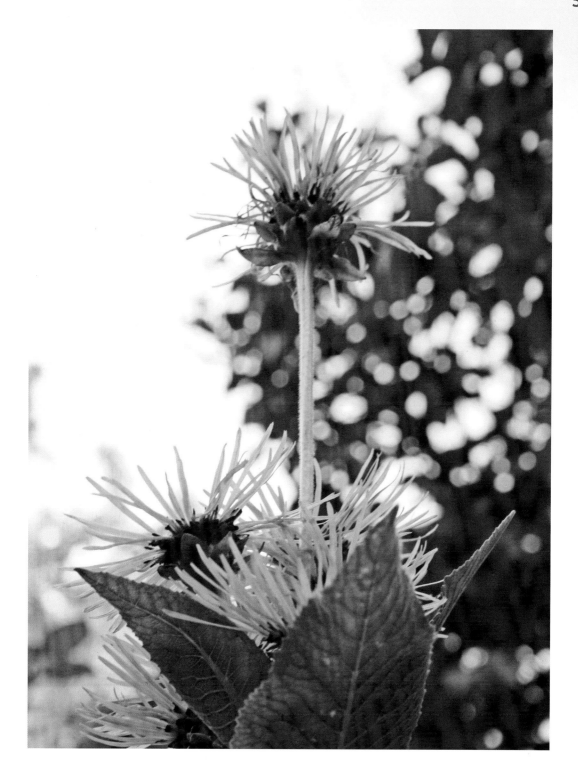

COMMON FUMITORY
Fumaria Officinalis
Contact with Our Ancestors

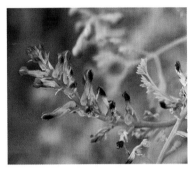

Common fumitory has been used as incense for a very long time, and the Germanic and Celtic peoples made incense from this wonderful plant. Fumitory was also called "elf smoke" and at that time was already a sought-after incense. The wise women and sorcerers of these peoples used the fumitory plant to contact their ancestors. It is also said that incense made with fumitory makes one invisible.

This does not mean that you will no longer be seen, but that a kind of protective shield will form around you, and the people or negative energies that want to harm you will lose interest in you. So be protected against witches and demons.

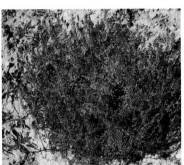

In earlier times, fumitory incense was burned to exorcise evil spirits. For this purpose, fumitory was grown in monastery gardens, so that the exorcists of the church always had this incense plant on hand. It could be compared with rue. This plant also played an important role in exorcism. In particular, rue incense is used against the evil eye.

After the incense ceremony, the windows of the room must be opened wide, so that the smoke can be carried outside.

WHERE AND WHEN TO GATHER

Fumitory loves sandy soil. Therefore, it is also often found in or near sandpits, but also along roadsides, where it is cut close to the ground. It is dried whole and chopped into small pieces for an incense.

This incense helps us against energy vampires. When we feel we are being drained by someone and realize that we are giving too much without questioning, a fumitory incense helps us find the golden mean again.

The plant spirit of the common fumitory shows us to again say NO.

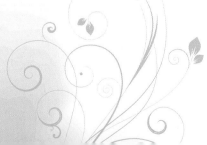

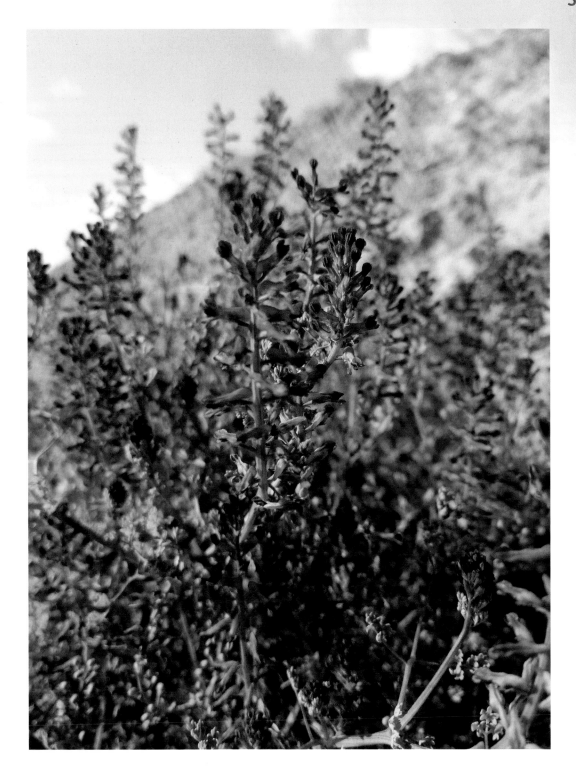

GOLDENROD
Solidago Virgaurea
Gives Us Light and Love

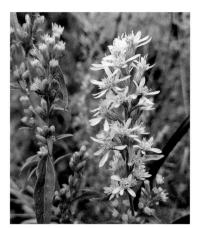

European goldenrod was burned as incense by the ancient Germanic peoples. In the seventeenth century, incense made from this plant was burned to drive away demons (illnesses), mainly in the case of communicable diseases.

A goldenrod incense is made to keep negative energies away from rooms. Because of its yellow color, it is one of the sun herbs, providing light and warming energies that strengthen our self-confidence. When used to treat partnership problems, this incense helps us think clearly again and slowly solve entrenched problems.

My personal experience is that burning incense as a sign of gratitude can be carried out very well with one made from goldenrod. For example, it is used when a test has been passed, one has recovered from an illness, or simply something has happened for which one is grateful. This is because the word "goldenrod" has its origins in folk belief and means a rod that shows one the gold. Gold is not intended to mean the metal gold, but the right way or just luck. When you have found the right way or experienced a great stroke of luck, you should show your gratitude by burning incense. The goldenrod also does good service for incense ceremonies that are carried out for augury or for money spells.

WHERE AND WHEN TO GATHER

Goldenrod likes to grow in old sandpits and fallow areas. It is collected from July to September. The entire plant is harvested a handbreadth above the ground and hung upside down to dry.

Burning goldenrod incense smells a little like honey. Goldenrod can also be combined with St. John's wort, marigold, amber, or mugwort roots to create an incense mix. The incense ingredients are dried before burning. You can use the European and also the American goldenrod, but the European is more authentic. The flowering herb is collected for making incense, meaning the flowers, stems, and leaves.

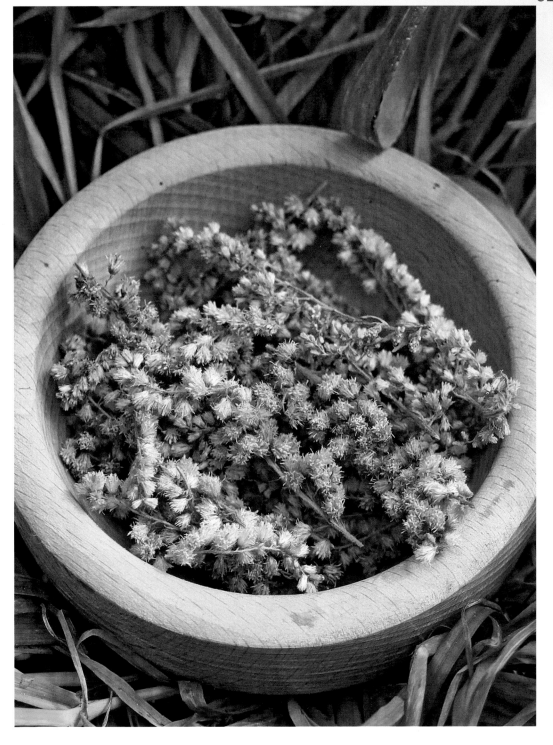

GROUND IVY

Glechoma Hederacea

Holds Interpersonal Relationships Together

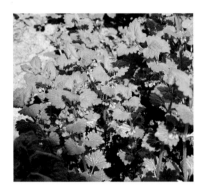

The ancient Germanic peoples burned ground ivy incense to bind their homes and property together and obtain protection. In earlier times, people placed wreathes of ground ivy on their heads in order to identify witches and bad people. This custom was widespread on Walpurgis Night.

In folk belief, ground ivy was regarded as a medicinal and magic plant. In the past, it saw widespread use in cattle sheds to protect the cattle against spells. To make ground ivy incense, use the dried stems, leaves, and flowers. It has an earthy and very pleasant scent. In Germany this wild herb is sometimes also called Gundelrebe, a feminine noun, which shows that features of both sexes can be seen in this plant. Dried ground ivy mixes wonderfully with angelica, ivy, and some larch resin to make a foretelling incense.

Burning ground ivy incense strengthens interpersonal relationships, such as family and also important friendships. This incense is effective for preventing harm and gives good energies the chance to take effect on us. A ground ivy incense bestows upon us clairvoyance, so that we can let our intuition run free, but also to avert dangers and damage from other people beforehand before they can strike us with full force. If you have a premonition, trust your gut feeling and believe that it will come. Mental hopelessness dissolves completely under the effect of this incense, and we acquire new courage and basic trust.

WHERE AND WHEN TO GATHER

Ground ivy is a creeping plant with small lilac-colored flowers. Its favorite place is right in the bushes, and that is where you will find it. It is collected almost all year round, except in winter.

This incense raises our spirit to a level that gives us the ability to prophesy. By burning ground ivy as incense, we develop instincts that reveal to us who wishes us ill.

Our intuition, our gut feeling, builds up until we become aware and rely on it.

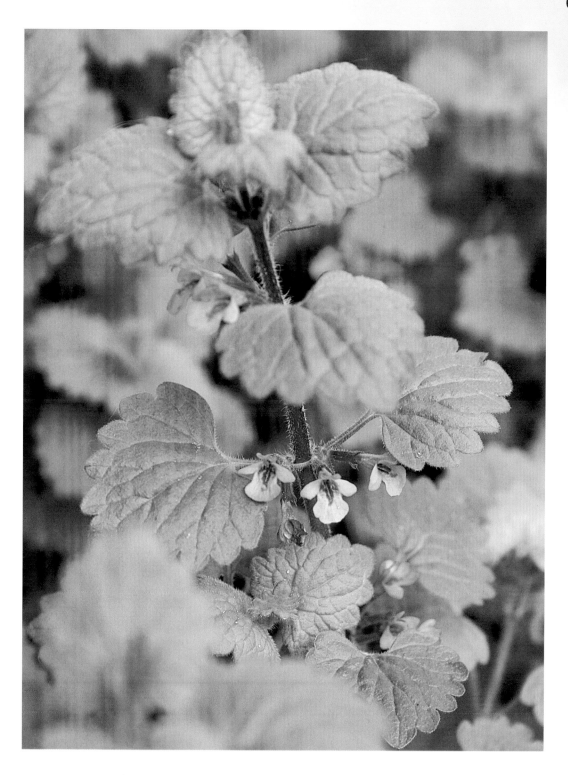

HOREHOUND

Marrubium Vulgare

A Great Protective Plant

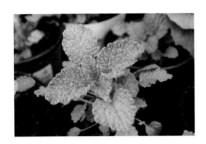

Our ancestors regarded the horehound as a great protective herb. Even the ancient peoples used it as a protective plant as well as in their rituals. They believed that when they burned incense made from this wild plant, the gate to the other world would be opened for them, and they would be protected at the same time. The ancient Wends used this herb to smoke out their houses when they wanted to shield them from curses. The horehound is a wild herb that has always been considered strongly repellent in folk belief.

Horehound was also immensely popular as an incense for cleansing houses, its smoke carrying any negative energy out the window. If you want to do such a house cleansing, you should first keep the windows closed for ten minutes, so that the negative energy can collect in the smoke and then escape with it through the open windows.

A horehound tea can be drunk before the burning of the incense. It promotes clear thinking, which is important when burning incense.

When we want someone to leave us alone, horehound is the incense of first choice. Its plant spirit is so powerful that it spreads a kind of invisible shield around us.

This makes us invisible to psychic attacks.

WHERE AND WHEN TO GATHER

This plant should not be gathered in the wild. Horehound is harvested at the time of the summer solstice because then, according to ancient knowledge, it should provide the greatest protection.

The horehound is rarely found in nature these days. I have never seen it in the wild myself. You can find it on fallow land where it is very dry. Unfortunately, horehound is protected and cannot be collected from the wild. Therefore, for this plant we should resort to stocks grown in the garden. However, there are also very good herbal pharmacies on the internet that have it in stock.

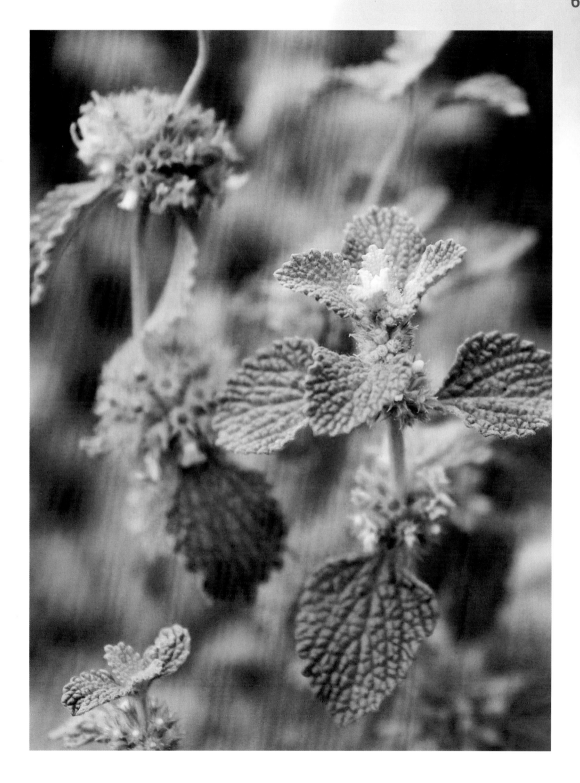

LADY'S MANTLE
Alchemilla Vulgaris
All in the Name of Women

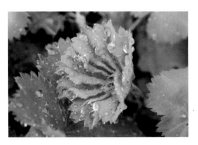

In incense lore, it is known that there are natural spirits in the lady's mantle, which massively support its plant spirit. In pagan belief the plant was dedicated to Frigg, a Germanic goddess who was regarded as the defender of motherhood and marriage and the guardian of the hearth and household.

Lady's mantle was also an essential part of an herb bundle that was burned in case of illness or to protect against lightning strikes. For these purposes it was collected with an herbal blessing. It also has a firm place in the belief in the magic number 9.

Lady's mantle was used by our ancestors as an incense against headaches of various kinds.

Lady's mantle incense was used primarily for women, but it can also be good for men who have too much aggression in them. This incense has a calming effect, and we see everything with serenity. It comforts women who are unsuccessfully attempting to become pregnant.

WHERE AND WHEN TO GATHER

In much of Europe, lady's mantle likes to grow in meadows and among low bushes; however, it does not grow wild in most of North America and must be cultivated. Its gathering time is from June to August. The leaves and flowers can be used for incense, and they are laid out individually for drying.

Even in the case of a miscarriage, the plant spirit of the lady's mantle gives us comfort and touches our soul. This warming comfort keeps us from despair and gives us hope when we might have already given up. We will feel relieved after this incense, free from grief and guilt.

Dried lady's mantle can be combined with yarrow, calendula marigold, and goldenrod to make an incense.

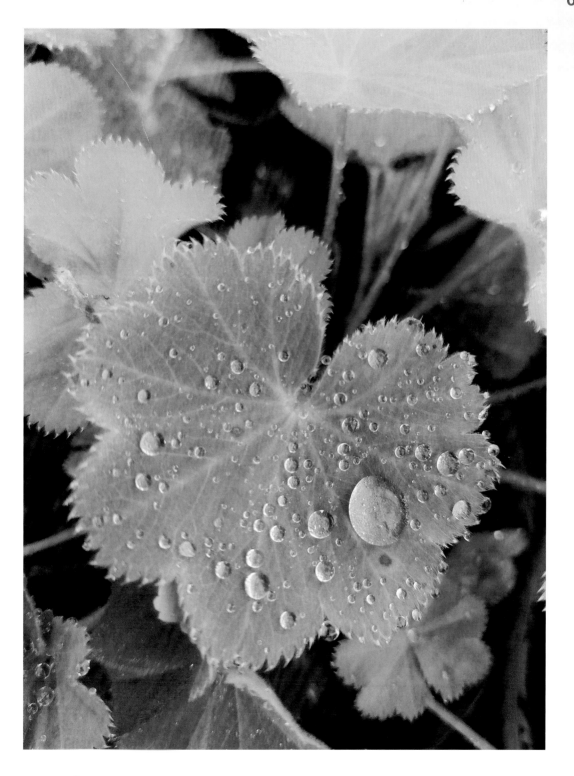

LAVENDER
Lavandula Officinalis

A Purifying Incense

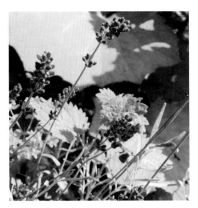

Burning lavender incense clears and cleans our mind. Smoke from the lavender has a calming and clarifying effect on our mind and body. As a result, embedded negative thoughts (evil spirits) evaporate, and we see more clearly into the present and future. Our soul world comes into balance, which is important for our well-being and health. As a result, we are in a more positive mood and ready to create something new.

It promotes inspiration and helps in our self-discovery. In a space where things are more hectic, you can burn lavender incense and immediately feel harmony, serenity, and calmness. In addition, this incense enhances our concentration, so we can focus on the essentials. Because the smoke has a cleansing effect, lavender can be used to treat houses or individual rooms where sick people have stayed or are staying. It purifies and disinfects the air. The dried flowers and leaves of the lavender plant are used for this purpose.

Lavender smoke has a floral and herbaceous scent; therefore, it is very popular in incense blends. Lavender harmonizes with pine needles or wood, mugwort, rosemary, and mint. I myself avoid mixing incense resins with lavender because they affect the smell, leaving little of the lavender scent. If you still want to smoke lavender with an incense resin, I can recommend larch resin, since its scent is not quite as intense.

WHERE AND WHEN TO GATHER

Lavender does no grow wild in most of North America (nor in Germany or much of Europe, except for in some Mediterranean regions), and therefore it must be purchased or grown in one's garden. Lavender should be cut in high summer. The day must be hot and sunny, since the plant develops its best qualities at that time.

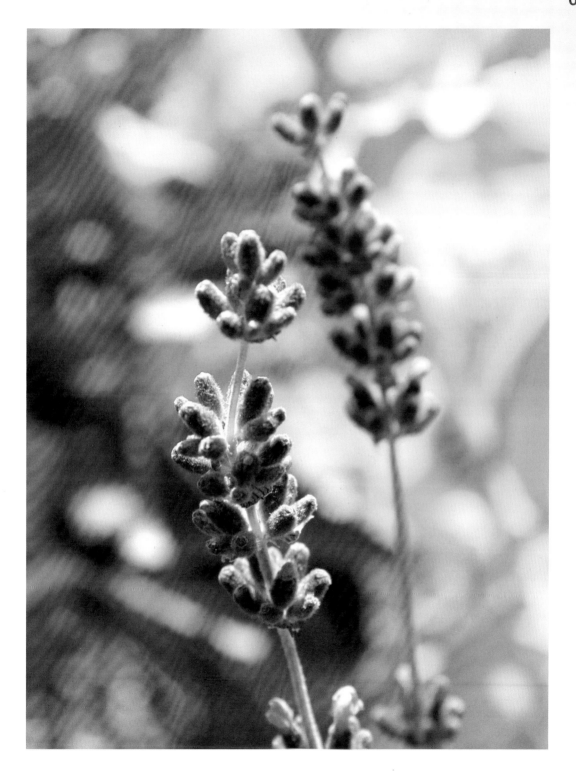

MARIGOLD

Calendula Officinalis

For Lucid and Truthful Dreams

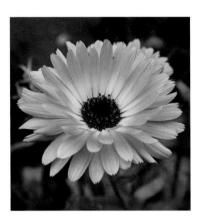

Lovers are exposed to smoke from burning marigolds to ensure that their love lasts forever. It brings sunshine into our hearts, and we become receptive to our counterpart. This incense also gives us a feeling of security, and we let beautiful old memories come back into our consciousness. This creates wonderful feelings that we know from the memories. This incense can also be used if one has pent-up emotional aggression. Our soul calms down and we come back into harmony with it.

In incense lore, burning marigolds as incense also stands for lucid and truthful dreams and intuition. To achieve lucid dreams, marigold blossoms are scattered under the bed, and marigold incense is burned before retiring. To fulfill wishes, a marigold tea should be drunk before going to sleep, and the bedroom purified with marigold incense.

We can sharpen our intuition with this plant. It is good for people who very often fall for the lies and intrigues of others. This incense strengthens people, enabling them to recognize dangers sooner and then remove them from their lives.

Marigold incense can be made using the whole dried herb or just the petals of the flowers. Smaller flower heads can be dried whole and burned. When burned, marigold incense produces an herbaceous scent.

WHERE AND WHEN TO GATHER

Marigolds are often found near fields in the northeast and western United States and adjacent parts of Canada as well as in many parts of Europe. For use in incense, this beautiful plant should be cultivated in the garden or pot-cultivated, because we never know whether wild plants near fields have been sprayed. Marigolds should be planted under a waxing moon around the summer solstice.

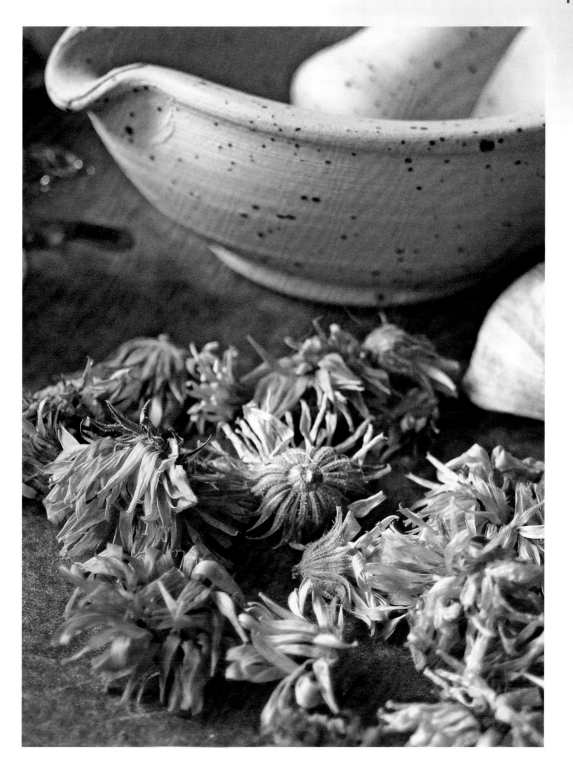

MINT

Mentha Sp.

Calms and Sharpens Our Mind

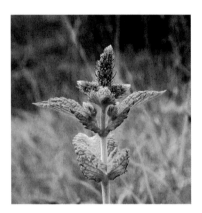

Burning mint incense calms and sharpens the mind at the same time. If we are ever plagued by lack of concentration, mint helps us get back on our feet. But mint incense is also a good choice for dealing with negative room energies. When we feel drained and very nervous, this incense calms us down and we can sit back, relax, and enjoy our existence. We see things more clearly, and our mind processes them better as a result. By using it we free ourselves from our self-made maze of thoughts and can solve problems about which we have thought too much and therefore found no solution. Its plant spirit gives us strength and clears our minds to perform new tasks.

The properties of mint incense range from healing, expelling, and clarifying to protective. Dried mint can therefore also be added to mixtures for protective incenses. In such incenses, the mint clears the air. That is why it is also suitable for smoking out old houses.

For this purpose, whole sprigs of mint are first soaked in salt water, and one then goes from room to room to sprinkle the purifying salt water. By sprinkling salt water, one cleanses the rooms of negative energies. We know such scenes from Christian customs when holy water is sprinkled.

Mint mixes well with lavender and rosemary to make an incense. The dried and crushed mint herb (stems and leaves, also flowers) is used for this purpose. Mints with a lot of menthol, such as peppermint, spearmint, or Spanish mint, are suitable for use as incense. Of course, domestic mints are best, such as the corn mint, pennyroyal, horse mint, and also water mint. So-called fruit mints with little menthol, such as the vine mint and the strawberry or banana mint, are not suitable for use in incense.

WHERE AND WHEN TO GATHER

Native mints are found in wild meadows, and the brook mint, as its name suggests, beside brooks. They are collected from May until the end of summer.

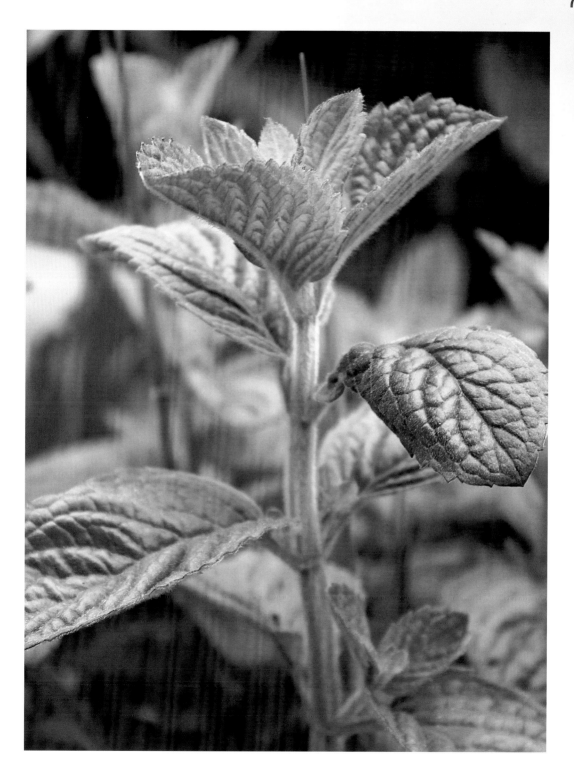

MISTLETOE

Viscum Album

The Mysterious One among the Incense Herbs

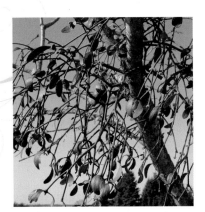

Burning incense made with mistletoe has a calming effect on our soul and expels negative energies from a house. It is a component of many protective incenses. If we want to escape from the hustle and bustle of everyday life, mistletoe is eminently suitable. Through it our soul comes to rest, and we have the opportunity to look inside ourselves and can complete our own soul journey. We will quickly realize what we want and what we would rather leave alone because it is not good for our soul. Sometimes we do not realize that our soul is suffering, because we are caught in such a daily routine and react only to external stimuli. This incense will accompany us to the roots of our soul to achieve inner contemplation.

Mistletoe incense is very suitable when we want to stand on the threshold between the otherworld and the present. This incense has long been used as a magical tool in ancestral invocation.

Mistletoe complements verbena to make an incense for winter evenings. Mistletoe incense gives off a slightly sweet, herbaceous scent.

WHERE AND WHEN TO GATHER

*European Mistletoe is found only rarely in North America, but a substitute, **Phoradendron leucarpum** (American mistletoe), is more abundant in the eastern half of the United States and in Mexico. Unfortunately, mistletoe often grows at the very tops of the trees, where it appears in autumn, when the tree sheds its leaves. After an autumn storm you should look there, because usually some do not hold and thus fall down. That's also how I always go to collect mistletoe.*

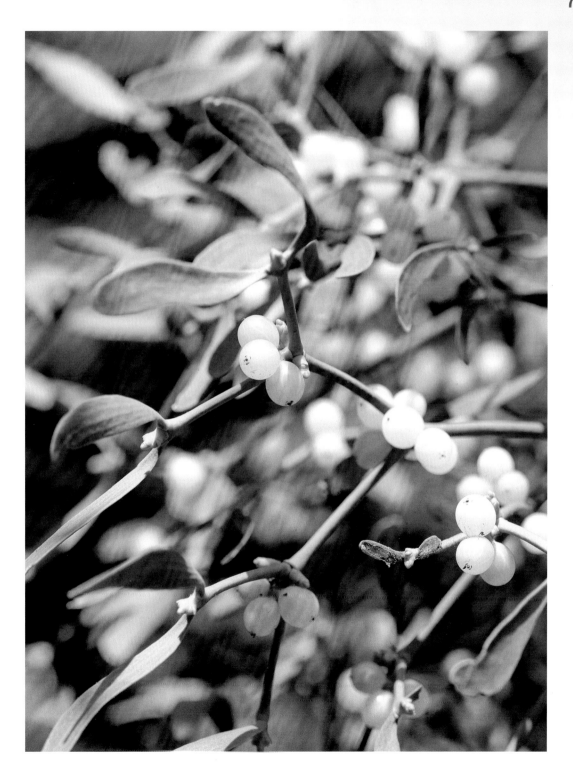

MUGWORT
Artemisia vulgaris

An Ancient Protective and Ritual Plant

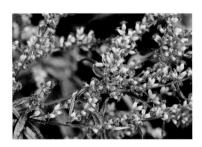

Mugwort drives away evil spirits. For our ancestors, this wild plant was a veritable must. Mugwort was dried, tied, and hung up everywhere, whether against witches, diseases, or storms. It was probably considered a very magic plant because of its aromatic scent. It was said to be hung in homes to ward off demons and the evil eye. Furthermore, it was taken against illnesses brought on by spells. When hung from the roof ridge, it provided protection against plagues and lightning strikes. In Denmark it was used to drive away the devil. Mugwort is also a component of the nine-herbs charm.

When unforeseen changes come into our lives, a mugwort incense provides powerful support. Also, when it comes to letting go after a separation or the death of a loved one, it promises us protection and support and helps us better cope with this process.

WHERE AND WHEN TO GATHER

Mugwort grows abundantly in much of North America (except for the southwest United States and Mexico) and in Europe, but especially on the edges of forests and paths, where it can be found in abundance. If you let it, it will also come into the garden on its own. Its harvesting time is from March to October. Its roots can be gathered all year round for incense.

Mugwort incense creates protection and warmth within us. When burned, mugwort gives off a strong, spicy, tangy plant scent that is said to enhance one's clairvoyant ability and ability to tell fortunes. Its relaxing and calming effect makes it well suited for an evening incense.

Mugwort also belongs in every incense mixture for use against negative energies during house cleansings.

For this purpose, an incense is often made from mugwort, rue, sage, juniper wood, and spruce resin.

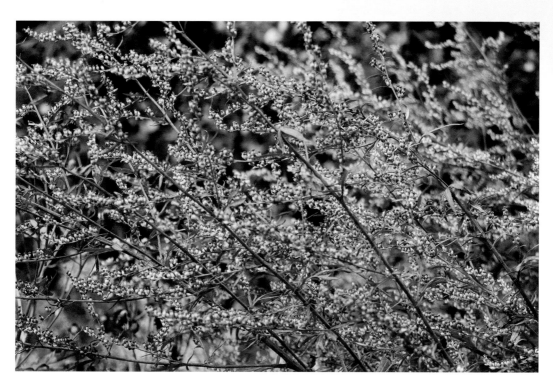

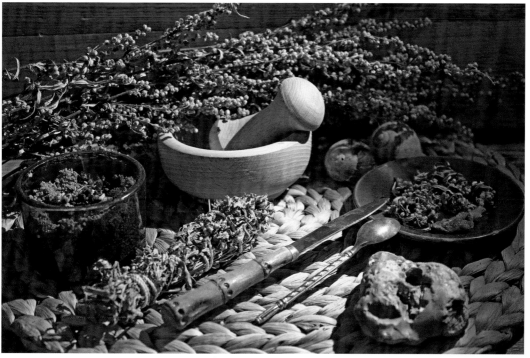

MULLEIN

Verbascum Thapsus

A Purifying Incense

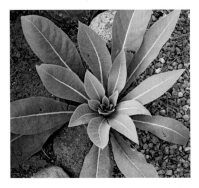

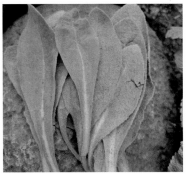

In early folk belief it was believed that burning mullein incense warded off black magic and demons, and it was regarded as a powerful agent against them. In the eighteenth and nineteenth centuries, mullein flowers were burned as incense to calm approaching storms and prevent lightning strikes. Incense made from mullein flowers and leaves was also burned in homes to rid them of mice.

Two hundred fifty years ago, women who suffered from excessively heavy menstruation were treated with smoke from burning mullein leaves. To do this they stood over the incense pan. In the old incense lore it was regarded as having protective, purifying, loving, cheering-up, healing, and also prophesying properties. I think that anyone who has ever stood in front of a mullein plant will be able to confirm this.

Every year I once again look forward to harvesting mullein and to drying and processing it into a wonderful incense. I wait for the right moment when it is in full bloom, because their flowers open at different times and fade very quickly. The plant's leaves can also be gathered and dried. They make wonderful tinder for an incense. In the past they were also used as wicks.

WHERE AND WHEN TO GATHER

Mullein can often be found in old sandpits or fallow land. They love this dry, sandy soil. Their collecting time is from July to September. The leaves, individual flowers, or the whole flower stalk are taken.

To purify one's karma, one can bathe oneself in the smoke from burning mullein. Before that, you should take a cleansing bath with mullein and possibly drink a tea made from the flowers.

Thus, one has cleared and purified his body. After this cleansing ceremony, the room must be aired out.

This incense is a true helper in unbearable times, to reduce overboiling emotions. We become calm and serene through its plant spirit and can avert many disputes. The scent of mullein incense is summery and honey-like. The mullein mixes well with roses and wild oregano to form an incense.

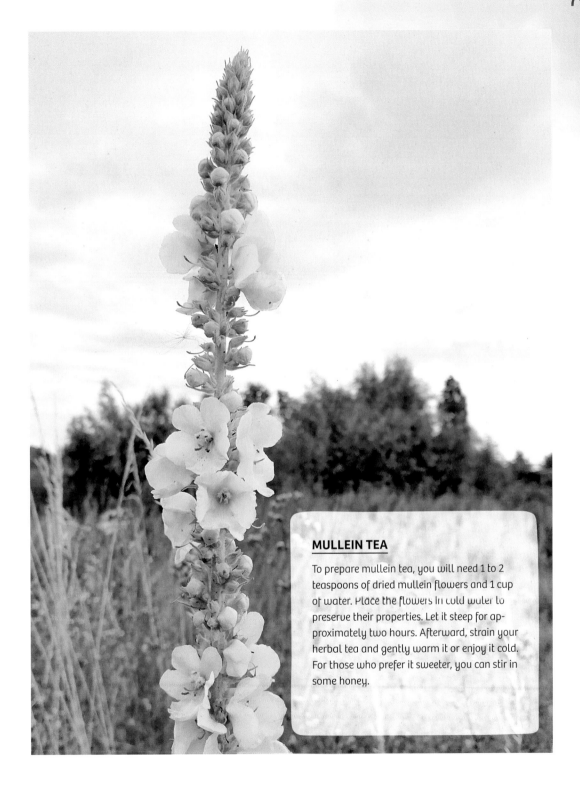

MULLEIN TEA

To prepare mullein tea, you will need 1 to 2 teaspoons of dried mullein flowers and 1 cup of water. Place the flowers in cold water to preserve their properties. Let it steep for approximately two hours. Afterward, strain your herbal tea and gently warm it or enjoy it cold. For those who prefer it sweeter, you can stir in some honey.

COMMON OREGANO
Origanum Vulgare
An Old Protective and Magic Plant

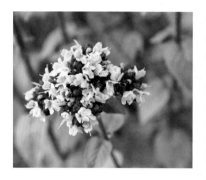

"Valerian, oregano, and dill—then the witch can't do what she wishes." A well-known saying of our ancestors, because oregano is a magic plant against sadness, bewitchment, and powerlessness. In former times it was spread about the house to protect the inhabitants from theft, witchcraft, and enchantment. Therefore, this plant is one of the occupational and invocation herbs because it protects against enchanted or transmitted diseases and curses. As well, smoke produced by burning oregano was used to cleanse the house and barn for protection against evil spells.

If you give this plant to a sad person, he becomes cheerful again. It has great value as part of an herb bundle. This plant was a vital ingredient in our ancestors' apotropaic powder (a powder against any harm; see page 44). According to old folk belief, it has a powerful plant spirit.

Burning incense made from this wild plant makes a person emotionally unassailable. It strengthens one's "personal power." To enhance the effect of an oregano incense, an oregano wine can be drunk before the ceremony.

To make this, mix 1 liter of red wine with 70 g of oregano flowers and let it steep covered for two weeks.

WHERE AND WHEN TO GATHER

If you want to gather wild oregano, you should look at the edges of fields or even in sandpits. There it usually grows abundantly. The oregano can be collected from June into the fall, bundled, and hung upside down to dry. It is easy to cultivate if it does not grow in your region.

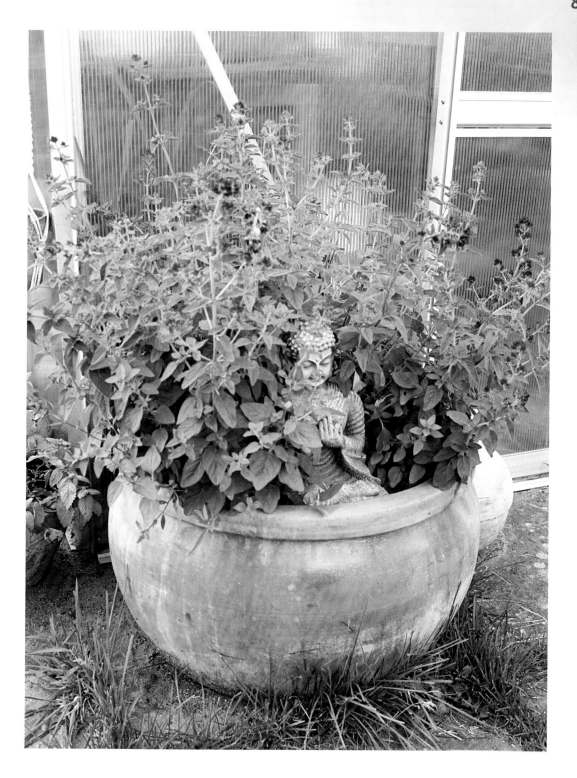

ROSE

Rosa Sp.

Giver of Self-Awareness

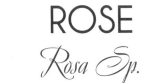

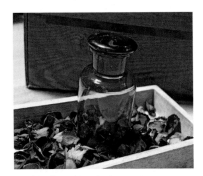

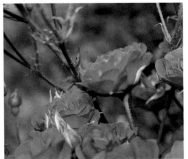

Incense made with roses takes away our depressive mood. Their plant spirit helps us let go of loved ones and restores inner peace with ourselves. This incense creates a gentle and peaceful atmosphere in which we can let ourselves fall. For people who are very jealous, incense with roses can do a lot of good. They can think more clearly about their jealousy and possibly recognize the reason for it and actively fight it. Jealousy blocks our life flow and is mostly superfluous.

Burning incense with roses enhances our inner balance and self-knowledge. Its plant spirit leads us, so to speak, out of this labyrinth of feelings again and puts us back on the path of our knowledge. The plant conveys love to us, also to ourselves. It shows us that we are loved, which enhances our basic trust. Burning rose incense is also helpful in dealing with partnership problems or for strengthening a partnership.

To strengthen a partnership, it is always recommended that the incense be burned in the bedroom, because this is the room where we share everything with our partner psychologically and physically.

WHERE AND WHEN TO GATHER

The petals of the rose are dried beforehand, loosely layered. You should collect rose petals for incense only from your own garden. If you know they have not been treated, then of course purchased roses can also be used. For my incense mixture I have planted some small shrub roses in a beautiful red. They bloom until November and sometimes even longer.

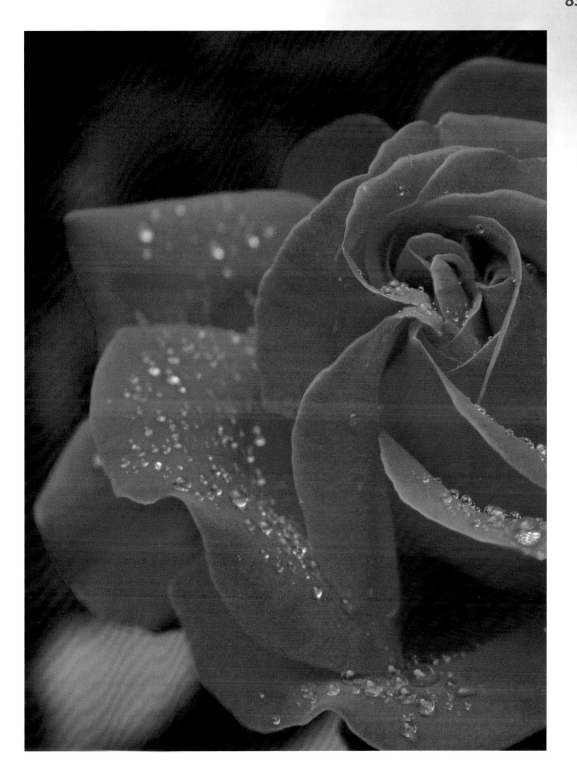

ROSEMARY
Rosmarinus Officinalis
For Parting and Transition

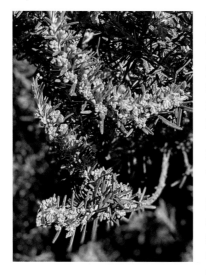

Rosemary is all about farewells and mourning. In incense lore it has healing, expelling, and purifying properties. Its plant spirit guides us through the labyrinth of mourning and parting. Its smoke contains strong cleansing energies. Rosemary is therefore suitable for smoking out houses. In the past, the rooms of the sick were smoked out with rosemary and juniper, in order speed up healing of the sick.

In the times of the plague, sickrooms and sick people were exposed to smoke produced by burning rosemary.

Rosemary can be burned as incense in cases of death, human or animal. This facilitates the transition of the soul. We can say goodbye and let go, which is important. Because if we do not let go, the souls of the deceased will not be able to part and will remain trapped. According to ancient folk belief, they then become revenants.

Burning rosemary incense is good for deadlocked problems, from which we sometimes cannot find the way out. The spirit of the plant will show us the way out and thereby clear our problems out of the way. This incense gives us strength, and we become aware of our inner strength and gain the courage to embark on new paths. Our mind also benefits from a rosemary incense; it becomes more lively and fresher and our concentration improves. This incense is quite suitable for anxious people. It reveals the self-confidence that lies deep within us, which can sometimes be hidden by self-doubt and fear. This incense is therefore perfect for problem-solving.

Rosemary is one of the very old incense plants. It is often used as a replacement for frankincense and mixes wonderfully with thyme to make a powerful incense.

WHERE AND WHEN TO GATHER

Unfortunately, rosemary does not grow wild in most of North America or in Germany (though it does grow in some European and African countries along the Mediterranean). It must be cultivated in one's garden or in a pot. We should harvest rosemary from June into August. Whole branches are gathered, which are then hung up and dried.

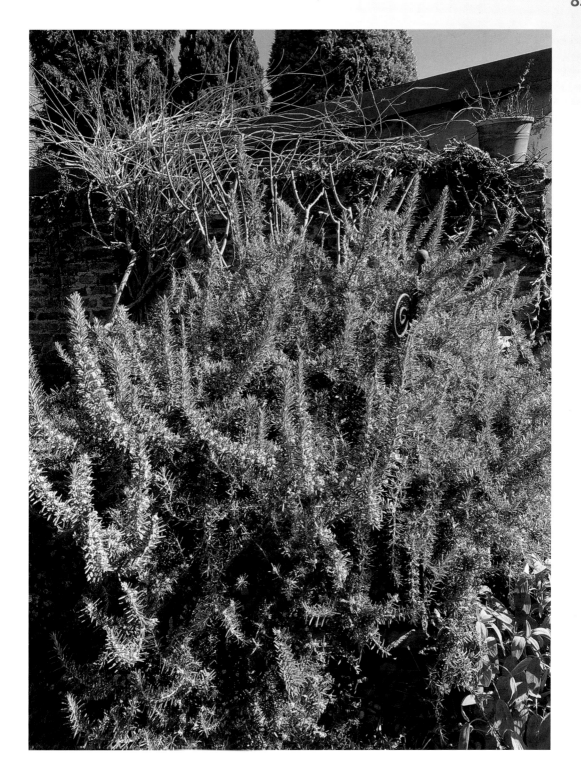

RUE
Ruta Graveolens

Protection against the Evil Eye

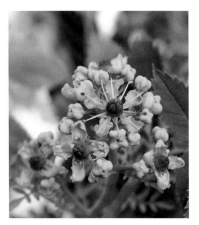

Burning incense containing rue against the evil eye dissolves curses and is strongly evil repellent. Perhaps someone talks badly about us, or things are said about us that are not true. There are also people who in their hearts wish us ill. These people pass on to us their negative energies, spells, curses, and everything that can adhere to us negatively. They usually have the evil eye. A rue incense helps us uncover so-called false friends in time.

Rue plays a significant role in Christian exorcism and was grown in monastery gardens specifically for this purpose.

At that time, people burned rue incense in their homes if they thought that they were haunted or that the the devil was up to no good. Today, this would be called negative or foreign energy. Rue is one of the protective herbs that protect against all kinds of bad things. But also, when one's mind is clouded, rue frees it and we get a clear view and find our way back to ourselves again.

This magic plant was also worn as an amulet, for protection against false accusations. For an incense that wards off harm, rue is combined with spruce resin, sage, rosemary, or tansy, or a combination of these.

WHERE AND WHEN TO GATHER

For use as incense, one gathers rue leaves, flowers, and seeds. Everything is loosely layered in a wooden tray to dry. Rue has a peculiar smell, which one has to get used to. It is harvested from the garden from spring until late summer. It is also naturalized to grow wild in a scattering of locations in the United States and Canada. Its small side shoots can be cut off, which are then bundled and hung upside down to dry.

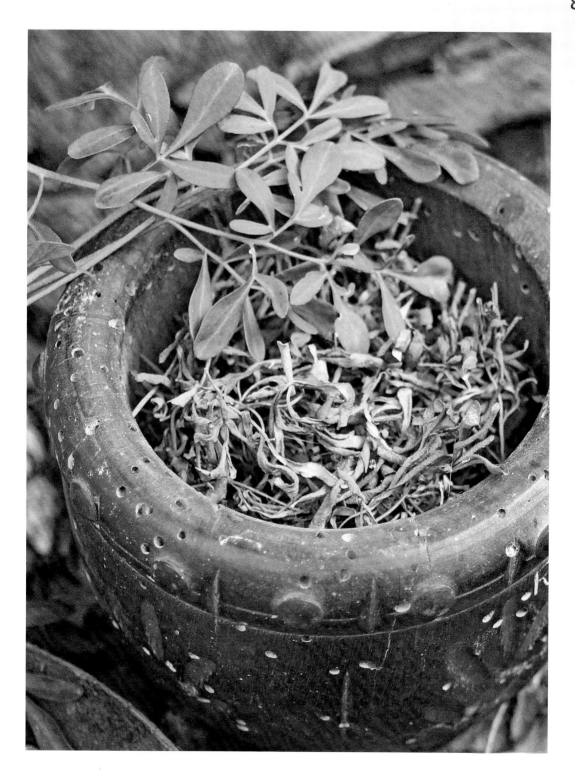

SAGE
Salvia Officinalis
Cleansing and Clarifying

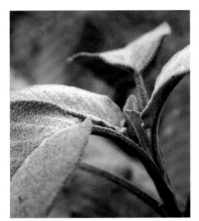

Burning sage has a clarifying effect on one's mind, purifying, protecting, expelling the negative, and healing, which is why it is an excellent and important incense plant. Sage incense cleanses the mind and soul and mentally opens all doors for us to rid old houses of negative energies. The best way to do this is to use an incense pan, like the ones used in medieval times to smoke out sickrooms. With an incense pan, one goes through the house from room to room, and from corner to corner. For it is in these places that negative energy resides.

Sage is also helpful in letting go of people; for example, in the case of a separation, death, or even a dispute. It makes one's mind clear and fresh, thereby enabling us to change our point of view. Our soul is rebuilt piece by piece. This incense is especially suitable for sensitive people, who often doubt themselves and lack confidence in their actions. Dried sage has a long tradition as an incense plant and magic remedy. In Turkey, sage was used to fumigate rooms in which the sick lay. It is one of the most popular incense plants. Sage mixes well with lavender, spruce resin, and rosemary to create a purifying incense.

WHERE AND WHEN TO GATHER

Sage grows wild in the southwestern United States and northwestern Mexico and in some of Europe. It is very easy to cultivate at home. Sage can be collected all year round. When drying sage, one must take care that the leaves do not touch one another; otherwise, there may be brown spots.

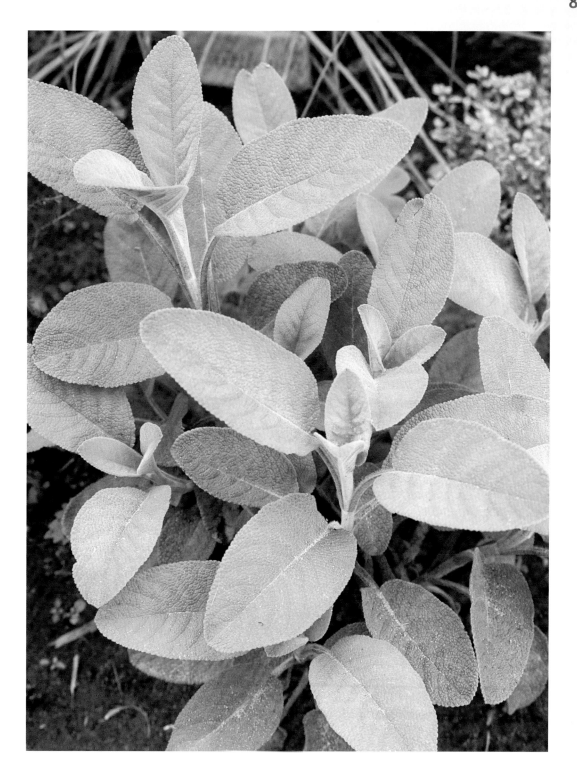

ST. JOHN'S WORT
Hypericum Perforatum

An Old Incense Herb

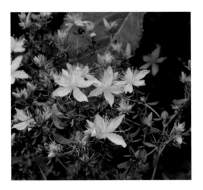

St. John's wort is one the ancient incense herbs used by our ancestors, and it has retained its magical properties to the present day. At the time of the summer solstice, St. John's wort was made into a belt, which was dried and then burned at the same time the following year, or burned as incense for protection from harm in the coming year. Exactly the same thing was done with mugwort.

During storms, St. John's wort was thrown onto the wood-stove or into the glowing coals. By doing this, people believed they were protected and that their home would be safe from damage, such as lightning strikes. In Havelland in Brunswick, people also spoke the following words:

"Is there no old woman who can pick St. John's wort now that the thunderstorm is gathering?"

St. John's wort was used to make "health incense," as our ancestors called it, and back then it had to be picked on a Thursday when the moon was waning. Folk belief often stressed that if it was to be used as incense, it had to be picked on June 24. I choose to collect St. John's wort right at the summer equinox, following the old tradition. The old folk beliefs said that it was precisely at that time that the plant's protective powers were at their greatest.

WHERE AND WHEN TO GATHER

St. John's wort can be found in meadows, field margins, and fallow land. This wild herb loves the sun. It is harvested a handbreadth above the ground between June and September. The whole plant is hung upside down to dry.

Today we burn St. John's wort incense to relieve tension. Such negative energies can enter into spaces where there is a lot of arguing. These spaces should always be treated with St. John's wort incense, so that the negative energies dissipate.

The plant spirit also shows us the proper way to get out of a period of depression. A St. John's wort incense strengthens us internally, and we are able to solve problems and find new ways. Anyone who wants to prepare his own incense should not ignore mugwort. St. John's wort can also be mixed with stinging nettle, goldenrod, and hazel wood.

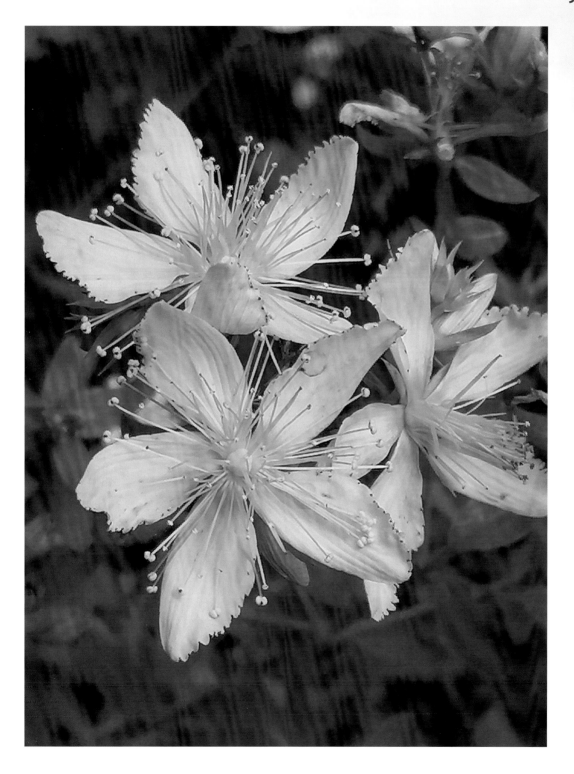

TANSY

Tanacetum Vulgare

Against Energy Vampires and Mischief

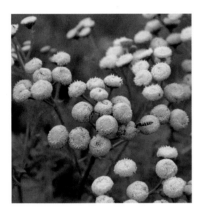

Burning incense with tansy has always been considered antidemonic and mischief repellent. Therefore, in incense lore it is used against energy vampires and impending disaster. In the past, witches and vampires were what we now see as energy vampires.

Burning tansy incense helps keep them at bay. It loosens up an aggressive environment and adds warmth of heart. It strengthens our self-confidence and nerves. Its plant spirit gives us vitality and strength on a physical as well as mental level.

In folklore, tansy incense was burned to prevent lightning strikes. For this purpose, the tansy can be burned together with mugwort, mullein, vervain, and St. John's wort.

It was one of the herbs used to make incense, along with rue, wormwood, elecampane, water astragalus, and valerian, which were collected and dried together on Ascension Day, August 15, to be used during incense-burning nights in the cattle shed and in the house against night spirits and witches. Whoever collects tansy at the witching hour on the night of the summer solstice and burns it as incense, and also carries small stalks of it with him, is said to be impervious to harmful spells.

WHERE AND WHEN TO GATHER

This wild herb can be gathered from July to September provided it is in full bloom, but the best time is late summer during a full moon. Tansy loves the edges of fields in full sun. There you will find it in abundance. Drying tansy is quite simple because you simply hang it upside down.

In earlier times, bundles of tansy were hung from windows and doors to keep mosquitoes and flies from entering. Tansy incense can also be burned to ward off these tiny pests.

Dried tansy mixes very well with mugwort and St. John's wort to form a protective incense. I usually also mix in a little pine resin.

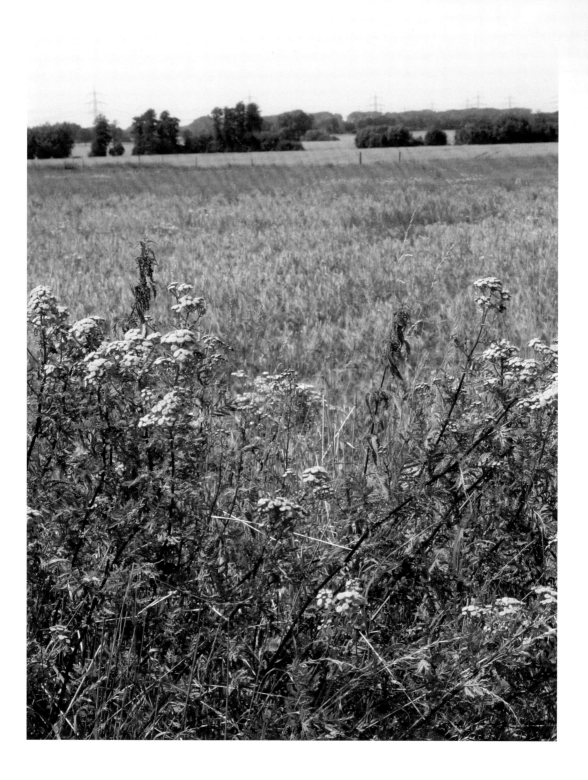

COMMON VALERIAN
Valeriana Officinalis
A Protective Herb for Our Spirit

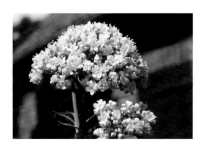

Valerian used to be called witchweed because it was believed that it could be used to dispel or repel hexes on humans and cattle. The evil eye was very much feared in earlier times, as were evil spirits (negative thoughts). An incense made from the roots of this plant dissolved everything into thin air. One also hung the whole plant over the door of the house, so that nothing negative could enter.

Nowadays, valerian is known for neutralizing our negative thoughts and giving us peace and inner reflection. It is a wonderful incense plant for the stormy winter months, when you have to deal with the winter blues more often. Valerian roots help us with nervousness and a stressful everyday life. Through the use of valerian incense, we come to rest and are able to relax, since it reduces mental stress. For this purpose, valerian roots can also be mixed with lavender and hops.

It is the roots of the plant that are usually collected; however, flowers and leaves can also be taken.

WHERE AND WHEN TO GATHER

Valerian is often found beside streams, since it likes areas that are slightly damp. Its flowering period is from July to August. Its flowers are harvested in summer, and its roots are harvested in autumn at the autumnal equinox. It is found in much of Europe and some of northeastern and northwestern North America.

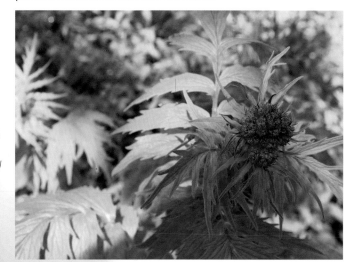

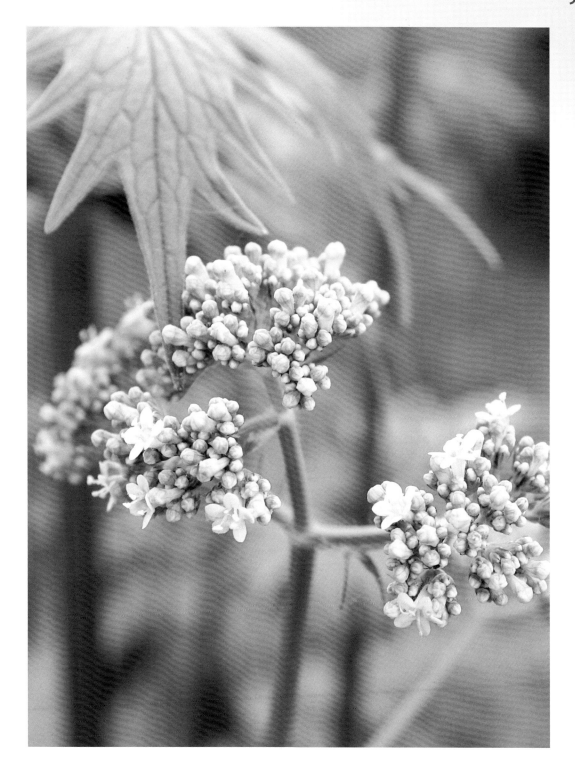

WILD FENNEL
Foeniculum Vulgare Var. Vulgare
Breaks Through the Sense of Loneliness

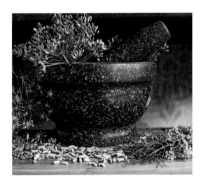

In earlier times, incense made from fennel was burned to protect one's home and possessions against evil spirits and negative energies. People who had been cursed with the evil eye had their curse removed by burning incense made from wild fennel. In earlier times, many intensely aromatic herbs were used to drive away all forms of evil. This probably had to do with the powerful smells of the various plants.

Fennel was also used to remove hexes. If someone was cursed, constantly ill, or pursued by bad luck, the person's curse was removed with wild fennel; for example, by bathing in water to which fennel was added. Everything about them that had been cursed entered the bathwater and was poured out with it. Thus, the person was freed. People who had been cursed or had a spell placed on them were also exposed to smoke produced by burning fennel.

Burning incense made from fennel gives us the feeling of breaking through the loneliness and looking inside ourselves. Loneliness and withdrawal usually come from unresolvable and pent-up emotions that a fennel incense releases. Its plant spirit helps us better classify our emotions and process them. It puts our feelings in order and has a stabilizing effect. Our nervousness leaves us and we see some things with different eyes. It enables us to breathe deeply and concentrate on the essentials.

Fennel incense gives off a sweet and earthy scent. The dried seeds, flowers, and also the leaves are used to make it. Fennel can be combined very well with coltsfoot, ground ivy, and lavender to make an incense. The seeds can be crushed a little before they are added. Everything else is crumbled.

WHERE AND WHEN TO GATHER

Wild fennel belongs to the Umbelliferae family, among which there are very many poisonous plants. Therefore, we should harvest fennel from our own garden or pot culture. Its flowers are harvested in summer, its seeds in autumn. The fennel flowers can be laid out to dry or hung up. The seeds are spread in a small oblong container.

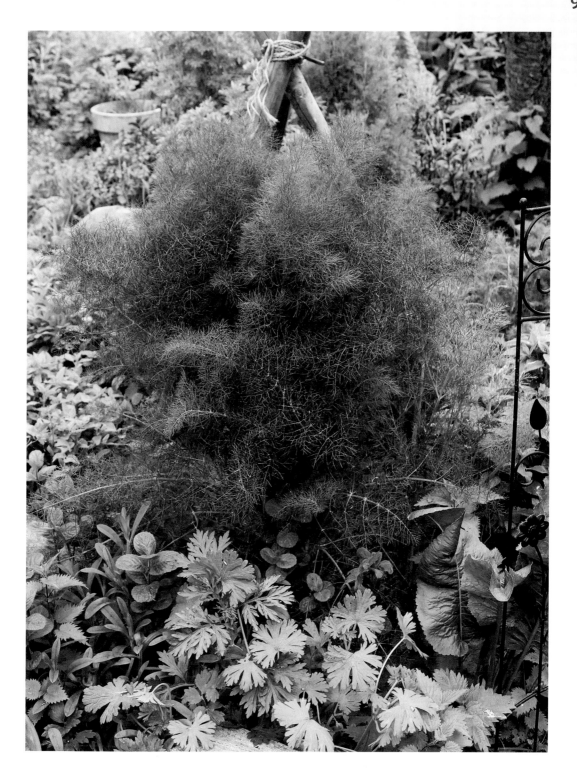

WILD HOPS
Humulus Lupulus
For a New Beginning and Restful Sleep

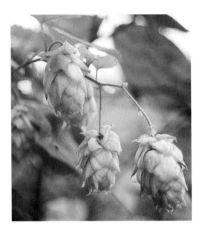

The process of using incense made from hops is less well known. Hops incense gives us strength to begin again in times of discouragement, and problems do not seem as bad as before. If one is experiencing overexcitability and the feeling that everything is too much, hops help achieve inner peace. The incense calms our nerves, and thereby we are able to get our well-deserved sleep.

Hops incense is recommended when one's body and spirit are experiencing stress and one is unable to turn it off. Burning hop incense is also useful when partners are quarreling, calming heated tempers.

Burning hop incense in the bedroom prior to retiring is recommended for a restful sleep with no bad dreams. To enhance its effect, a small pillowcase can be filled with hop cones. The hop's plant spirit gives us a restful sleep.

Dried hop cones are well suited to an incense mixture with lavender and rose petals. This incense is gentle and designed for sensitive people. Its plant spirit is very benign.

WHERE AND WHEN TO GATHER

The hop is a climbing plant and grows mostly at the edges of forests. There you can find it abundantly from late summer until autumn. This is when its hop glands are at their most mature. When you gather the hops, you must be careful that the yellow hop glands do not fall out when you pick them. It is best to harvest with a larger paper bag into which the cones fall directly when picked.

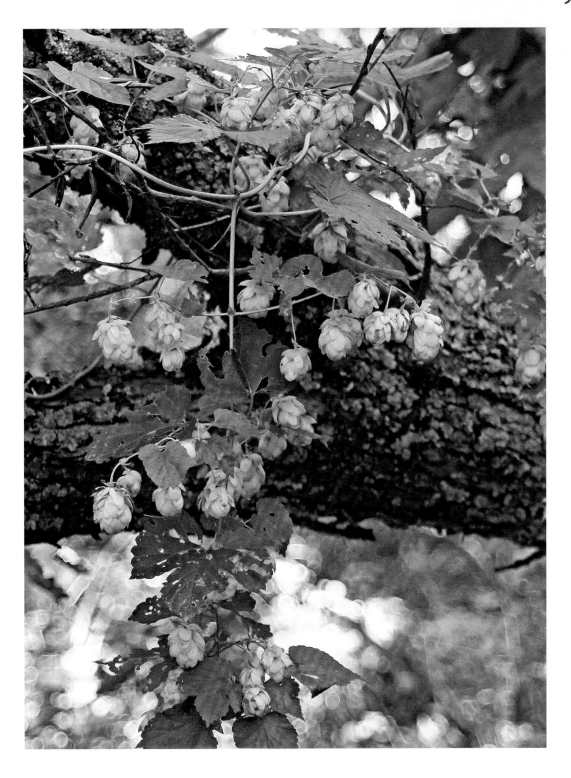

WOODRUFF
Gallium Odoratum

Protective and Helpful

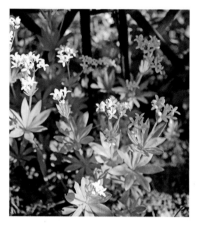

Unfortunately, the practice of using woodruff as an incense has been largely forgotten. Anyone who has a hectic everyday life can achieve deep relaxation in the evening by burning woodruff incense, provided that they can let go and leave everything behind them. It is an incense for inner contemplation and great peace. Simply let your soul unwind is the message that this beautiful forest plant wants to convey to us.

Our ancestors burned woodruff as incense to support women during childbirth and to protect the newborn child from the evil eye. Burning woodruff incense was considered to have a strong witch-repellent effect. In general, it was known to repel all evil from a person. Woodruff incense was burned for recovery in sickrooms and also as a defensive incense to ward off any disease demons.

Its properties in incense lore are protective, victorious, helping, and healing.

In folklore, the woodruff is an old forest mother, who protects lost children in the forest. From this we see that this plant is one of the protective herbs.

For use in an incense, the aboveground parts of the plant are dried along with the flowers. During the drying process, you have to make sure that your collected material does not turn brown. To prevent this, I put the woodruff in a shallow wicker basket and cover it with a linen cloth.

Woodruff mixes well with peppermint, resins, and St. John's wort. In the past, woodruff was not cultivated in gardens; instead it was collected in the deep forest. A strong incense can be made from woodruff, pennyroyal, and St. John's wort. To clear your head and get a fresh breeze in the house, you can use an incense consisting of thyme, woodruff, and juniper.

WHERE AND WHEN TO GATHER

As its name suggests, the woodruff's home is the forest, but it can also be found in gardens in shady places. It can be cultivated without problems. In the forest it very much likes rather lighter places. Its unmistakable smell becomes apparent only when it dries. If it is to be used in incense, the best time to gather woodruff is from Walpurgis Night until August. It grows in many European regions and is naturalized in some locations in the United States and Canada.

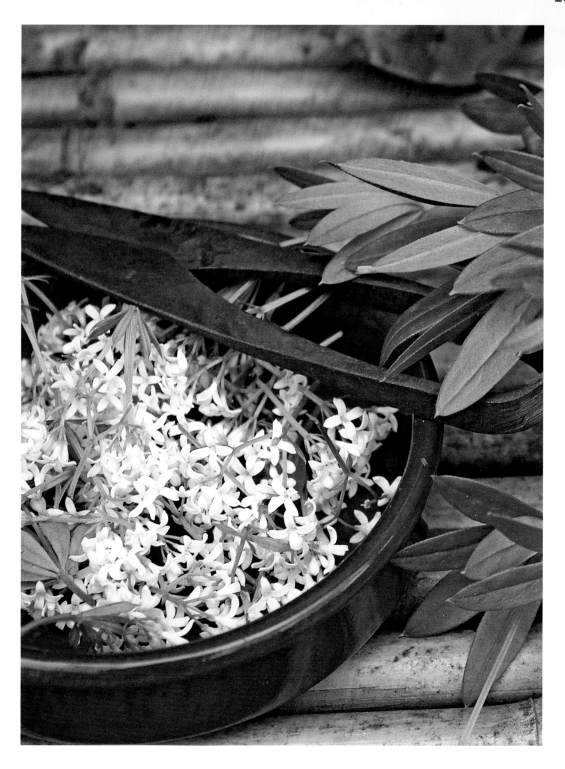

COMMON WORMWOOD
Artemisia Absinthium

Defense against Illnesses

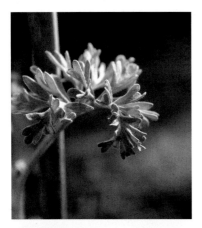

In early times, wormwood was used as a protective incense; for example, to ward off the evil eye. As well, at Christmas and New Year's Eve it was burned in the home for protection against spells. During the Middle Ages, if an illness broke out in the cowshed and got out of hand, it was purified with an incense mixture of wormwood, juniper, oregano, pennyroyal, spruce resin, and rue. As one can see, wormwood was and is a protective plant. This is due to the pervasive smell that it gives off.

Burning incense with wormwood gets our life energy going again. It carries our soul out of the darkness, and through it we come out of the labyrinth of hopelessness and again see a light at the end of the dark tunnel. We escape the melancholy and can again grasp clear thoughts. A wormwood incense gives us strength and enables us to avoid being distracted by negative thoughts and instead find the proper path.

To the ancient Slavs, wormwood was antidemonic. When hail threatened, they put wormwood on the hearth fire. In folklore, the mother's bed, which held her and her newborn, was purified with wormwood incense to protect the child from the evil eye. In the past, dried wormwood was also used against flies and mosquitoes, but also against bad smells and diseases. Therefore, the wormwood was very popular as an incense even in times of plague, when it was usually mixed with juniper needles or even twigs.

This plant has a very strong odor of its own, which not everyone likes. Wormwood mixes wonderfully with fumitory, juniper, and yarrow. If you are thinking about planting wormwood in your garden, note that it spreads quickly.

WHERE AND WHEN TO GATHER

Wormwood should be gathered in the late summer. By then, having been exposed to full sun, it has stored up all of its good qualities.

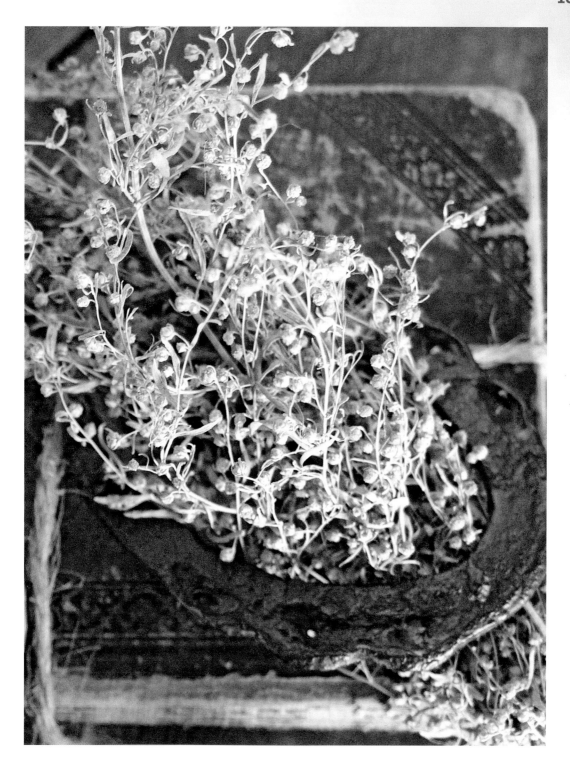

YARROW
Achillea Millefolium

Spiritual Helper for Our Soul

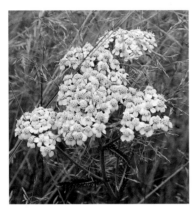

When we burn yarrow incense, it helps us establish a mental and physical balance. The message of yarrow is

Moral Attention and Mental Justice.

If we have had a sad experience or even a very drastic realization, a yarrow incense is the helper of our soul.

Through the plant spirit we regain courage, determination, and self-confidence, which has fallen by the wayside.

Thus, we see what we have experienced in a more relaxed way, take it into ourselves, and process it positively. We now see it as a positive experience and understand how we can perhaps learn from it. Anyone who would like to feel it a little more intensively can prepare a yarrow tea before the incense ceremony and drink it in sips. Thereby one becomes very relaxed and feels in harmony with nature.

Incense with yarrow is perfect for dissolving negative energies in houses.

In incense lore, the properties of yarrow incense range from healing, exorcising, and prophesying to loving. Its smoke was also used to purify objects.

WHERE AND WHEN TO GATHER

Just like tansy, yarrow loves to stand in full sun at the edges of fields. It is also best gathered at the time of the summer solstice—that is, in June, when its flowers have just opened. When harvesting, make sure that you cut the plant a hand width above the ground, because its stem is very firm. Otherwise, when you pick it, you will pull out the whole plant with the root. To dry yarrow, hang it upside down.

The whole dried herb is used for a yarrow incense. After gathering yarrow, hang the entire plant upside down to dry. Yarrow mixes well with wormwood and marigold.

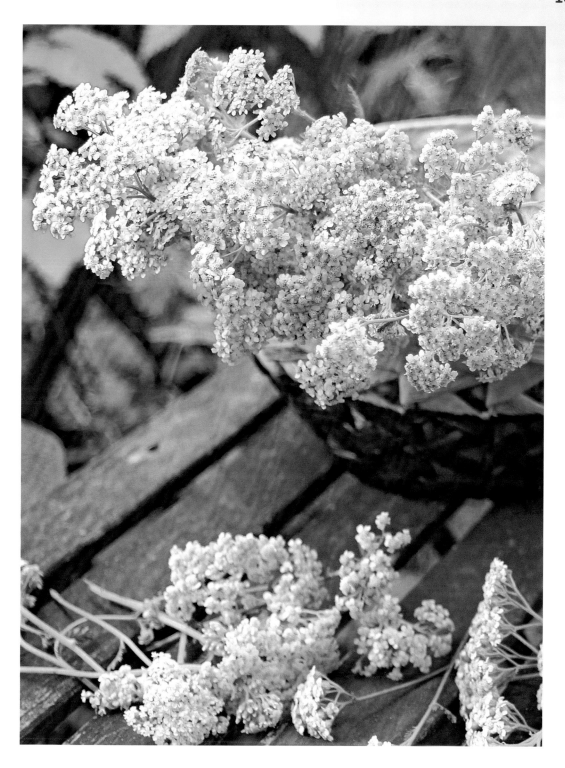

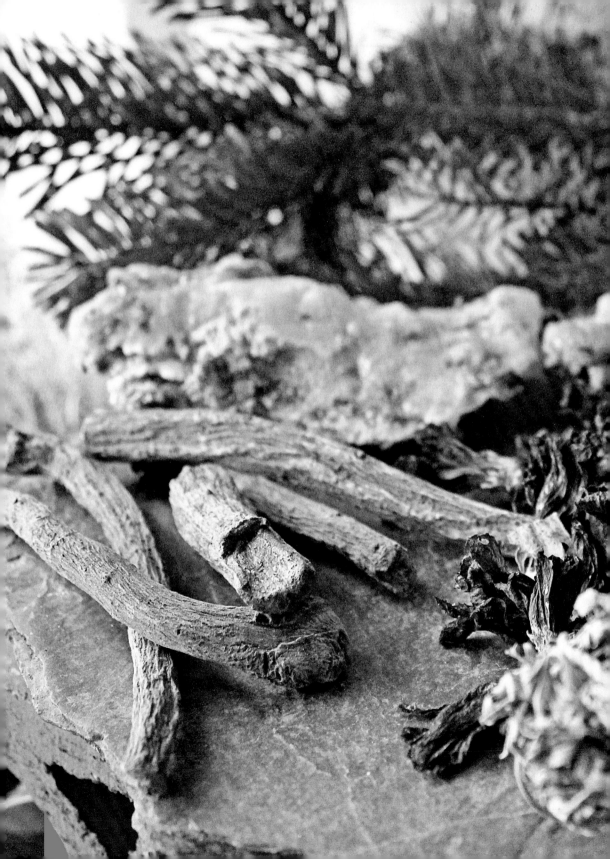

BURNING INCENSE MADE FROM WOODS AND RESINS

Personally I prefer to burn woods and resins. Coniferous wood impregnated with resin is a wonderful incense experience on cold, still winter evenings. Just like that, with a good book, warm and cozy, and a hot drink, with the smell of the incense as it crackles next to you. A blessing for our psyche in this digitalized world. And don't forget to turn off your cell phone!

Many of our trees donate their wood to provide incense. The juniper is one of the oldest incense plants and had great importance in folk belief. According to ancient beliefs, a juniper had to grow to the left of the front door, so that no one could come in who would think badly of us. Coniferous trees such as spruce or larch give us their lovely fragrant resin, which even has a germicidal effect.

BIRCH
Betula Pendula

Sign of a New Beginning

Incense made with birch awakens new energies in us and causes our stream of life to flow again. We are free for new tasks and also carry them out precisely. We are ready for a new beginning. A birch incense drives away our "winter blues" and nips negative thoughts in the bud. So, we feel light and exhilarated and can pull ourselves together for fresh deeds. This incense promotes our creativity. But the birch also helps with hardened problems in relationships, because its plant spirit loosens this hardening, and we can again look to the future with our partner.

Because the birch has a strong cleansing power, during incense ceremonies, exorcisms, or enchantments the participants were first "beaten" with birch branches, so that the evil in them clung to the branches and could then be thrown into the cleansing fire. This fire was fueled by birch and brushwood. Afterward the birch incense ceremony was conducted. In incense lore the birch also played a key role in Walpurgis Night.

Many plants, including the birch, have proven themselves useful in protective incenses. Birch is also one of the protective herbs. It has a protective and expelling energy. The broom at the front door, famous in folklore and believed to have magical power to ward off evil, had to be tied with birch twigs.

The birch mixes well with hawthorn and mallow flowers to make an incense. If desired, some larch resin can also be added. All parts of the birch can be used in incense, such as birchwood, bark, small twigs, and the leaves.

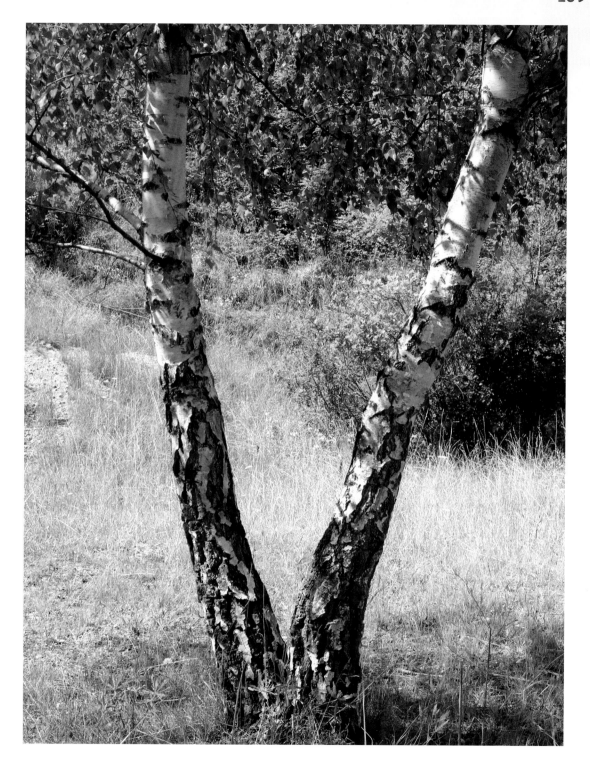

CRABAPPLE

Malus Sylvestrus

Especially for Love Incenses

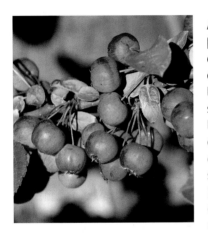

Apple trees have long been used to make love incenses. If, for example, a relationship is no longer working the way we envisioned it, an incense made from apple seeds is a suitable choice. It brings two loving souls back together again, even if they have drifted apart, so that they can once again understand and respect each other. This incense is also highly effective when we are seeking a new life partner. If we meet someone, it makes us attractive and self-confident. Because beauty and love come from within, and this is exactly what the plant spirit of the apple tree wants to convey to us: that we radiate from the inside out, and that we should not pay attention to a person's appearance. The apple incense detaches us from a material way of thinking and makes our heart radiate.

Burning incense made from the apple tree keeps away witches and devils. Applewood is also part of the belief in the magic number 9. In early folk belief, people bathed in nine kinds of fruitwood to wash away black magic that had been conjured up, and poured it out with the bathwater. In incense lore it is regarded as foretelling, healing, and loving. It was believed that one could achieve fertility or immortality by burning apple incense. To the Celts, the crabapple, a native apple tree, was one of the seven sacred trees. Crabapple trees were also thought of as oracle trees, with which one could foretell the time of one's death.

The bark, seeds, and wood of the apple tree mix well with spruce resin and roses to create an incense. You can also use small pieces of dried apple.

The crabapple should be chosen for incense because it grows wild and is native to many regions. Nowadays they often grow beside dirt roads. The fruit of these apple trees is small, hard, and extremely sour if one bites into it.

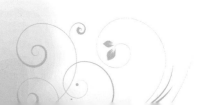

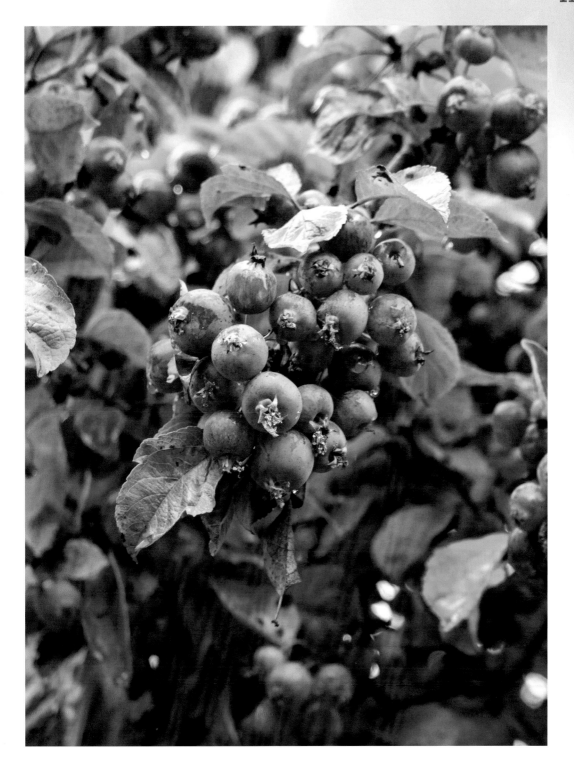

EUROPEAN HORSE CHESTNUT
Aesculus Hippocastanum
Counteracting Narcissism in Our Environment

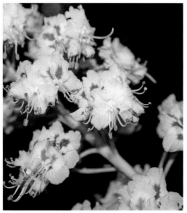

Burning incense made from the horse chestnut provides vigor and strength when we have reached a tired point in our lives. It clears our head and gives uplift to our soul.

This is exactly right for the beginning of autumn. Through this incense we obtain inner wealth and can happily and calmly walk through our lives.

The horse chestnut came to Germany only in the middle of the sixteenth century (it can also be found in other parts of Europe and in parts of northeastern and northwestern North America) and has quickly established itself in folk belief as a healing, lucky, and protective tree. Therefore, we should use these three properties of the horse chestnut in incense lore; for example, to give our thoughts healing vibrations. Because sometimes we cannot escape from our "thought vortex," incense with parts of the horse chestnut can help us find the way out of this situation.

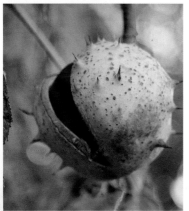

Burning incense made from horse chestnut protects us and helps us maintain our cheerfulness and self-love. We are thus protected from possible manipulation from the outside, especially by energy vampires and narcissistic people. If we are aware of this, we can purify ourselves with horse chestnut incense before meeting such people.

You can use the tree's wood, bark, fruit, leaves, and flowers to make a chestnut incense. Scrape the bark from a small branch with a knife. The well-dried wood you can plane to obtain small pieces. The flowers should be dried on a piece of linen, because otherwise they can stick to the surface during drying. This is also why they need to be turned over frequently when drying, or you can hang them upside down. Horse chestnut blends wonderfully with beech, birch, and oak to make an incense.

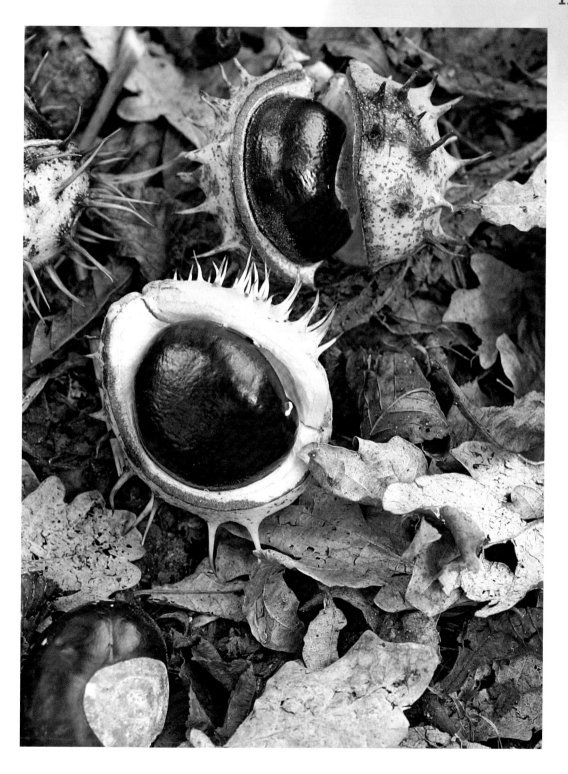

EUROPEAN LARCH
Larix Decidua
Giver of Self-Confidence

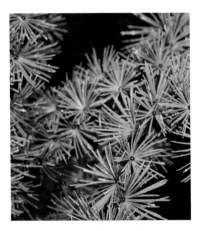

Burning incense made from the larch helps us make a new beginning. It gives us the self-confidence that we sometimes lack to reshape our lives. For many people, doubt gnaws at their self-confidence, and they fear that they may not be able to do something. This hinders them from creating or tackling new things. An incense made from the larch takes away the doubt, so that we can take a step forward. We obtain the missing courage and also the assertiveness that is important to reach our goals.

Even when we may want to part with people who accompany us on our life path, a larch incense is a good companion. It protects us on this path from negative foreign influences, and it acts like a shield. This incense makes us happy and content, so that we can harmonize mind, body, and soul. Larch has a strong protective plant spirit, which teaches us how to protect ourselves from all kinds of harmful spells. It makes us sensitive to such negative energies, so that we can detect them before they can do us harm.

To burn incense with larch, you can use the resin, bark, twigs, needles, and also the resinous cones. However, larch is protected or endangered in much of North America and should therefore be left alone there: check with local regulations wherever you are. Larch resin should be stored for two years prior to use in order to obtain its beneficial properties. Also, its fragrance is then much sweeter, and it does not smoke so much when burned. The larch mixes wonderfully with nettle, tansy, moss, and fern to create an incense.

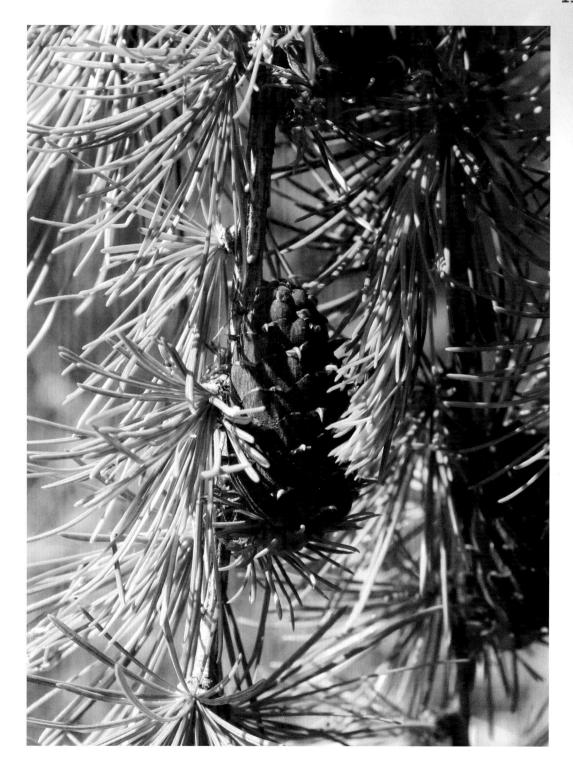

HAWTHORN
Crataegus Sp.
Strengthens Our Sense of Togetherness

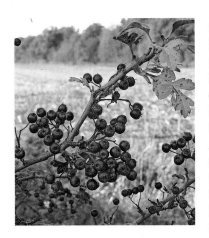

Burning hawthorn is a part of ancient incense lore. People have always believed that the hawthorn possesses the powerful plant spirit of healing and magic trees. Therefore, it also symbolizes the keeping away of negative energies in our environment. Its wood has played a role in magic since time immemorial; for example, when discussing water. A hawthorn wood stopper was used to close a water bottle. An old belief also says that you can keep a hawthorn in the garden, because it prevents the entry of evil spirits. This wood protects against thunderstorms and lightning. In former times, hawthorns were decorated with strips of cloth, woolen threads, human hair, and even small gifts, because it was believed that they encouraged the spirits of nature in the hawthorn to do good for the inhabitants of the house.

To burn incense with hawthorn gives us back the sense of togetherness. In some people it has truly been lost. For people with a narcissistic streak, this incense is the accompanying way to possibly get out of their behavior, as long as this trait is known to them and disturbs them. The plant spirit of the hawthorn shows these people that the sense of togetherness is something wonderful, because giving is more beautiful than taking.

If you want to burn hawthorn incense, you can use the dried flowers, leaves, fruits, and wood. The respective smoking ingredients must be crushed beforehand. The dried hawthorn wood can be scraped or planed. Hawthorn blends pleasantly with dried elderflowers, blackberry leaves, sloe wood, rose hips, and hazelnut leaves to a powerful incense.

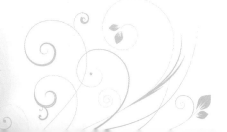

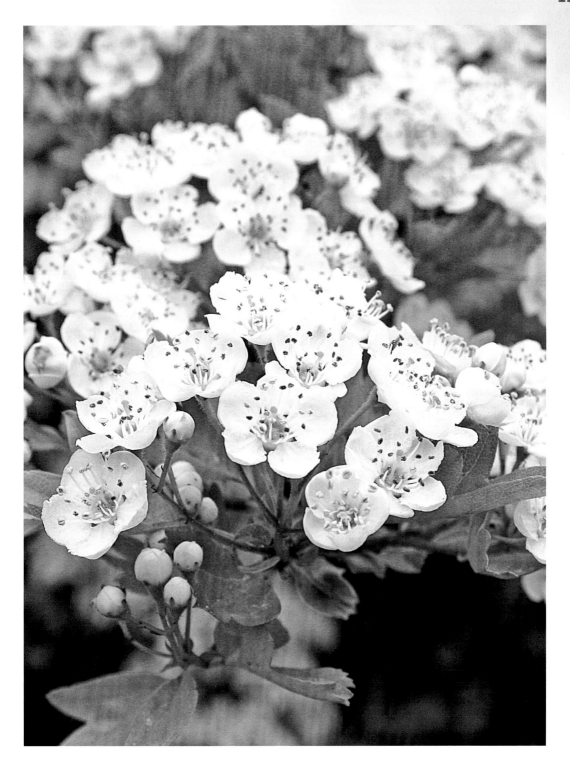

HAZEL

Corylus

Home of the Spirits of Nature

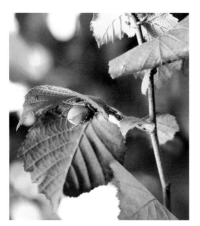

The ancient Germanic tribes used the hazel in their ceremonies to pacify their gods. It was especially important to them, as well as the elder and the rowan. In them dwelt the spirits of the house, which protected their homes and property. In pre-Christian times, the hazel was associated with the cult of the ancestors. This shrub was considered a symbol of spring and immortality because it carried the germ of life of a new plant.

A hazel incense gives us mental strength, especially in interpersonal matters. The plant spirit bestows adaptability on us. It gives our soul the meaning of its existence and gives us back the associated cheerfulness. This incense has a strong effect on our sexuality, causing a love that has fallen asleep to be awakened to life.

A hazel incense has a slightly sweet scent. Rose petals and juniper wood go wonderfully with hazel incense. Of course, it must be laid out in layers and dried before use.

WHERE AND WHEN TO GATHER
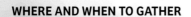

Hazel leaves or wood should be collected in the fall, shortly before the hazel bush loses its leaves. Hazel bushes like to grow at the edges of fields.

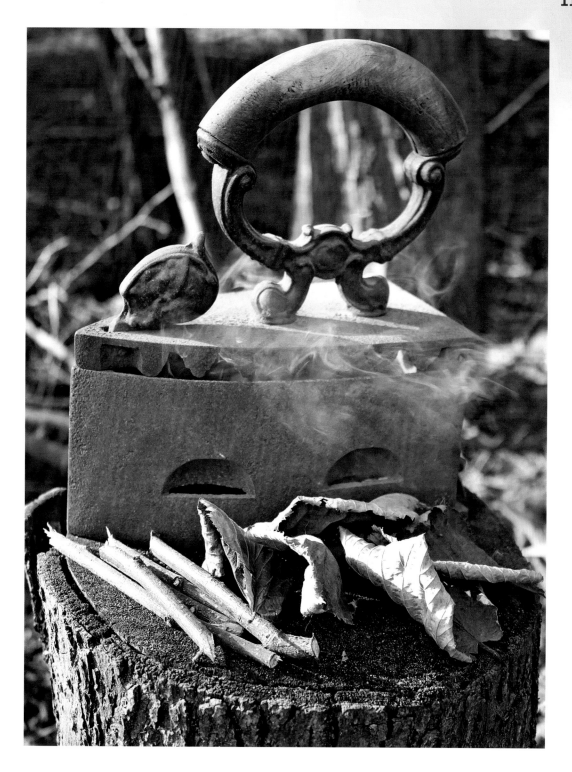

JUNIPER

Juniperus Communis

Experience Pure Magic

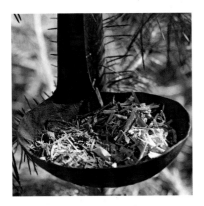

Before you start looking for a juniper, I would like to stress that juniper is a protected species in many regions, so it should be left alone as per local regulations. A juniper incense is one of the great protective incenses. It is believed that people in the Stone Age had already come into contact with juniper as incense. From the Middle Ages until well into modern times, people used juniper incense against plague epidemics. Juniper berries were carried on glowing coals in incense pans through the sickrooms. It has retained its magic powers until today. Juniper berries were smoked to ward off evil, since juniper has always been considered protective and guarding against negative energies. The plant spirit also helps wandering souls find their way home. It keeps people's envy away and drives away witches and demons and the diseases and curses they conjure up. Juniper is one of the very old incense plants.

This incense strengthens our inner shield, which is sometimes lost due to many events. The spirit of the juniper helps us rebuild it.

Juniper's plant spirit gives us courage to tackle new things. It gives strength and confidence and helps let go of emotions that are addictive. An incense with juniper wood cleanses the emotional world when you have gotten bad vibes from other people. Juniper strengthens our attention, makes our mind alert, and is even said to give us the gift of prophecy.

Juniper incenses are especially well suited for charging people and spaces with new life energy. The berries, needles, and branch tips are used. Juniper gives off a fragrant smoke.

It mixes well with pine needles, moss, and oak leaves to make an incense.

BURNING THE INCENSE

To use juniper incense, take 1 tablespoon of crushed juniper berries and put them on the glowing incense charcoal. Now carry the censer from room to room, not forgetting the corners, and smoke out the rooms. This cleans the air and is effective against colds.

Leave the smoke in the room for a while and then you can let it out of the window. This incense can be burned up to three times a week to get negative energies out of the house.

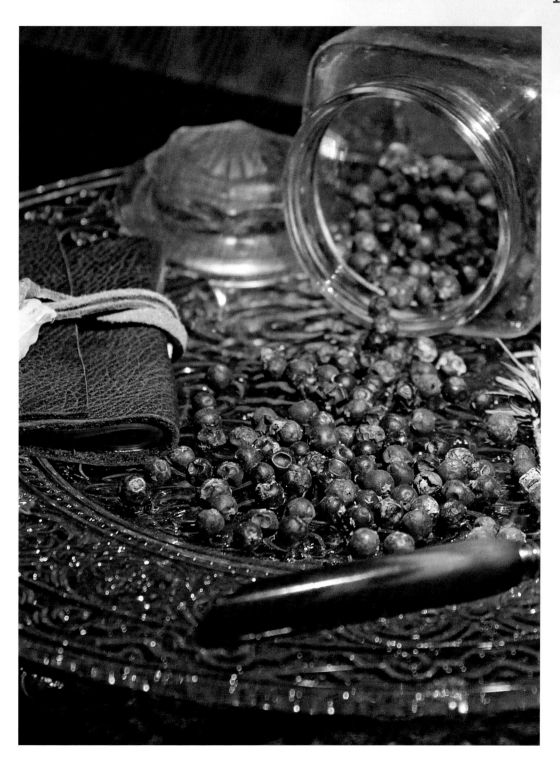

SPRUCE RESIN

Incense of the Poor

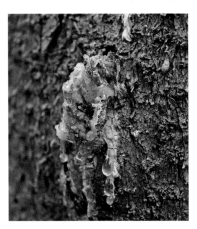

In earlier times, incense was difficult to obtain or was unaffordable for most people, and therefore spruce resin was used as a substitute. Hence the names "forest incense" or "incense of the poor." The spruce's needles, wood, and resin can be used as incense.

Because of their scent, in earlier times tree resins were used in purification and disinfection ceremonies as a remedy against the epidemics of the time, as they were during cold season, beginning roughly in autumn, to relieve the symptoms of the afflicted. Spruce resin has a germicidal effect and can therefore disinfect the air in the room. Spruce resin is also used to cleanse houses from bad energies. If you have the certainty or even just a suspicion that a person is speaking ill of you, you can burn spruce resin. This will invalidate this unwanted foreign energy, bring it to a standstill, and possibly send it back to its originator. Also, when moving to a new house, the individual rooms should be smoked out with spruce resin, so that everything old dissolves, freeing space for the new.

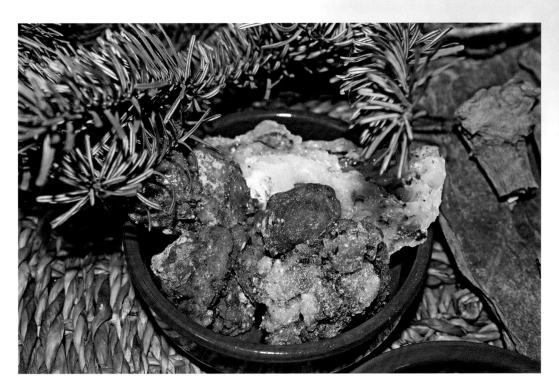

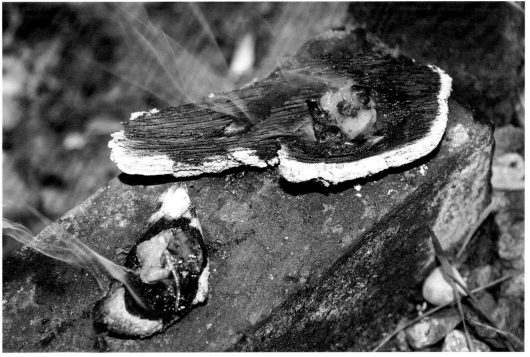

WHITE WILLOW
Salix Alba

Pathbreaking and Encouraging

Burning willow wood incense helps us find the right path in different phases of life and the right point in important decisions. The plant spirit gives us a straightforward skill, so that we decide for the right thing. But also, if our soul has arrived at a very dark point, a willow-wood incense cheers us up again. It takes the darkness from our soul and lets a light at the end of the tunnel shine for us. We then only have to take the path toward the light to reach the right decisions.

Its plant spirit gives us protection on this path, and we do not let anyone talk us into anything. Some people do not begrudge us the path to happiness, and we can also get rid of that through the positive energies of this incense. At the same time, the incense made from the willow promotes the earth connection and also causes our fears to disappear.

We no longer have to decide between yes and no but will know from the beginning what we want.

Burning willow wood strengthens our self-confidence. In the past, people burned willow branches to ward off lightning strikes and violent storms, and for this they used the hearth fire.

Dried willow wood mixes wonderfully with ivy, boxwood, oak wood, and spruce resin to create a directional incense. Willow bark and leaves can also be used, but the wood has the best properties for incense. Please take willow wood and bark only if you can find some on the ground.

From younger branches you can scrape off the bark with a knife, so it can be dried better. Chop the peeled branches and let them dry as well.

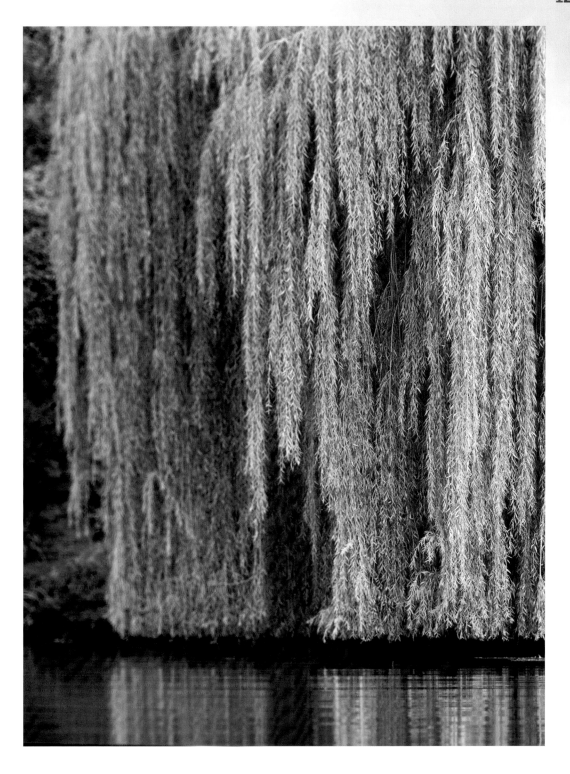

INDEX